Zero Effort Technologies

Considerations, Challenges, and Use in Health, Wellness, and Rehabilitation

Synthesis Lectures on Assistive, Rehabilitative, and Health-Preserving Technologies

Editor
Ronald M. Baecker, *University of Toronto*

Advances in medicine allow us to live longer, despite the assaults on our bodies from war, environmental damage, and natural disasters. The result is that many of us survive for years or decades with increasing difficulties in tasks such as seeing, hearing, moving, planning, remembering, and communicating.

This series provides current state-of-the-art overviews of key topics in the burgeoning field of assistive technologies. We take a broad view of this field, giving attention not only to prosthetics that compensate for impaired capabilities, but to methods for rehabilitating or restoring function, as well as protective interventions that enable individuals to be healthy for longer periods of time throughout the lifespan. Our emphasis is in the role of information and communications technologies in prosthetics, rehabilitation, and disease prevention.

Zero Effort Technologies: Considerations, Challenges, and Use in Health, Wellness, and Rehabilitation
Alex Mihailidis, Jennifer Boger, Jesse Hoey, and Tizneem Jiancaro
2011

Design and the Digital Divide: Insights from 40 Years in Computer Support for Older and Disabled People
Alan F. Newell
2011

Copyright © 2011 by Morgan & Claypool

All rights reserved. No part of this publication may be reproduced, stored in a retrieval system, or transmitted in any form or by any means—electronic, mechanical, photocopy, recording, or any other except for brief quotations in printed reviews, without the prior permission of the publisher.

Zero Effort Technologies: Considerations, Challenges, and Use in Health, Wellness, and Rehabilitation

Alex Mihailidis, Jennifer Boger, Jesse Hoey, and Tizneem Jiancaro

www.morganclaypool.com

ISBN: 9781608455195   paperback
ISBN: 9781608455201   ebook

DOI 10.2200/S00380ED1V01Y201108ARH002

A Publication in the Morgan & Claypool Publishers series
SYNTHESIS LECTURES ON ASSISTIVE, REHABILITATIVE, AND HEALTH-PRESERVING TECHNOLOGIES

Lecture #2
Series Editor: Ronald M. Baecker, *University of Toronto*
Series ISSN
Synthesis Lectures on Assistive, Rehabilitative, and Health-Preserving Technologies
Print 2162-7258   Electronic 2162-7266

Zero Effort Technologies
Considerations, Challenges, and Use in Health, Wellness, and Rehabilitation

Alex Mihailidis
University of Toronto

Jennifer Boger
University of Toronto

Jesse Hoey
University of Waterloo

Tizneem Jiancaro
University of Toronto

SYNTHESIS LECTURES ON ASSISTIVE, REHABILITATIVE, AND HEALTH-PRESERVING TECHNOLOGIES #2

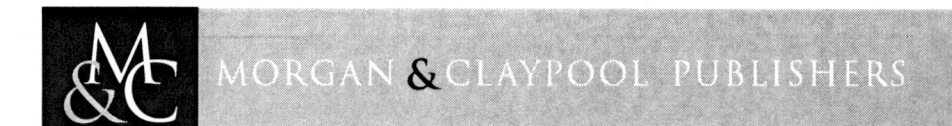

MORGAN & CLAYPOOL PUBLISHERS

ABSTRACT

This book introduces *zero-effort technologies* (ZETs), an emerging class of technology that requires little or no effort from the people who use it. ZETs use advanced techniques, such as computer vision, sensor fusion, decision-making and planning, and machine learning to autonomously operate through the collection, analysis, and application of data about the user and his/her context. This book gives an overview of ZETs, presents concepts in the development of pervasive intelligent technologies and environments for health and rehabilitation, along with an in-depth discussion of the design principles that this approach entails. The book concludes with a discussion of specific ZETs that have applied these design principles with the goal of ensuring the safety and well-being of the people who use them, such as older adults with dementia and provides thoughts regarding future directions of the field.

KEYWORDS

Zero-Effort Technologies (ZETs), pervasive computing, artificial intelligence, disability, health, rehabilitation, wellness

Contents

Preface ix

Acknowledgments xi

1 Lecture Overview 1

2 Introduction to Zero Effort Technologies 3
   2.1 What is a ZET? 3
   2.2 Overview of Pervasive Computing 6
       2.2.1 Pervasive Computing Principles 6
       2.2.2 Elements of Pervasive Computing Systems 9
   2.3 Overview of AI Principles 12
       2.3.1 Commonly Used Sensing Techniques 13
       2.3.2 Commonly Used Machine Learning Approaches 16
       2.3.3 Modeling Interactions Between Users and ZETs 21

3 Designing ZETs 27
   3.1 Common Design Paradigms 27
       3.1.1 Universal Design 28
       3.1.2 User Centred Design 30
       3.1.3 Incorporating Privacy in the Design Process 32
   3.2 Key Design Criteria for ZETs 36
       3.2.1 Develop for Real-World Contexts 37
       3.2.2 Complement Existing Abilities 37
       3.2.3 Use Appropriate and Intuitive Interfaces 38
       3.2.4 Encourage Involvement with the Users' Environment 39
       3.2.5 Support the Caregiver 39
       3.2.6 Complement each Individual's Capabilities and Needs 40
       3.2.7 Protect the Users' Privacy and Enable Control over Preferences 40
       3.2.8 Ensure Expandability and Compatibility 40

4 Building and Evaluating ZETs ... 43
- 4.1 In Silico Testing ... 43
- 4.2 Benchtop Trials ... 44
- 4.3 Actor Simulations ... 45
- 4.4 Trials with Clinical Populations ... 46

5 Examples of ZETs ... 47
- 5.1 Areas of Application ... 47
- 5.2 Overview and Comparison of Examples ... 48
- 5.3 Autominder ... 48
- 5.4 The COACH ... 54
- 5.5 Archipel ... 57
- 5.6 Assisted Cognition Project ... 58
- 5.7 PEAT ... 59
- 5.8 PROACT ... 61
- 5.9 ePAD ... 62
- 5.10 The HELPER ... 64
- 5.11 Rehabilitation Robotics ... 66

6 Conclusions and Future Directions ... 69
- 6.1 Limitations of ZETs ... 69
- 6.2 Future Challenges and Considerations ... 70

References ... 73

Authors' Biographies ... 81

Preface

Since the early 1980s there has been a growing area of research that focuses on the use of technology to help mitigate the effects of various health conditions, and to help improve the outcomes of rehabilitation. These technologies have ranged from simple reminding devices to help with medication management to advanced robotic systems that can help people recover lost motor, sensory, and cognitive functions. Over these years, this area of work has been given many different labels and definitions including cognitive assistive technology, cognitive prostheses, cognitive orthotics, quality of life technologies, and more recently ambient assistive living technologies. No matter the label or definition though, all of these technologies have something in common: they have been designed to help specific users to achieve functions that they would normally not be able to achieve.

In order to be effective, appropriate, and accepted solutions, assistive technologies should be able to provide support without increasing the workload of the user or other stakeholders, such as caregivers and clinicians. However, more often than not this goal has not been achieved and as a result the majority of these devices have been abandoned by their users. In response, researchers and others involved in this field have started to recognize the need for more usable devices that can only be developed with direct input from end users. Researchers have also recognized the need for more advanced techniques to be used in the development of these technologies that help to reduce the need for explicit user input and interactions.

Significant advances in fields such as computer science and biomedical engineering are allowing imagination to be turned into reality; incorporating advances such as artificial intelligence is greatly reducing, and in some instances eliminating, the amount of effort required to operate technology. As this trend towards little or no required effort gains momentum, the bounds of what can be achieved with new technologies for healthcare and rehabilitation continues to expand. This includes the application of sophisticated artificial intelligence and sensing algorithms that, in the past, have only been used in more constrained problem spaces, and the involvement of various disciplines, such as computer science, that are traditionally not involved in healthcare and rehabilitation. It is these continuing trends that will help to further advance this field, and that will enable new, cutting-edge technologies to be developed to continue to support users with their healthcare and rehabilitation needs.

Alex Mihailidis, Jennifer Boger, Jesse Hoey, and Tizneem Jiancaro
August 2011

Acknowledgments

Parts of the materials presented in this book have been reproduced from a chapter previously written by the authors with permission from IOS Press and the Associated Editors.

Alex Mihailidis, Jennifer Boger, Jesse Hoey, and Tizneem Jiancaro
August 2011

CHAPTER 1

Lecture Overview

The intersections and collaborations between the fields of computer science, biomedical engineering, and assistive technology are rapidly expanding, causing dramatic increases in the capabilities of intelligent systems for supporting healthcare and rehabilitation. As the applications of these devices become more pervasive and complex, it is important that these new technologies are designed in a way that best serves the people that will use and rely on them. This becomes even more important when these technologies are intended for people with one or more disabilities, such as people with mobility, sensory, or cognitive impairments. The special needs of these populations mean they require special considerations throughout the design process as the technologies may be relied on to support a person's well-being. This is especially true in the development of advanced artificially intelligent technologies for supporting health and rehabilitation applications as these systems require additional resources and data to ensure that they accurately represent the users for which they were developed, and that they operate in a reliable fashion. Typically, these additional requirements are addressed through high levels of involvement of the end user in the development, training, and usage of these systems. However, this is not always a reasonable expectation of special populations.

This lecture introduces *zero-effort technologies* (ZETs). A ZET is a new class of technology that uses advanced computer-based techniques, such as computer vision, sensor fusion, decision-making and planning, and machine learning to autonomously operate through the collection, analysis, and application of data. This capability enables ZETs to autonomously learn about users and their environments, enabling them to support the well-being of users with little or no effort from the users. As such, while ZETs are useful and usable by all populations, they are especially appropriate for people who are not necessarily able to reliably or explicitly provide input as would be required from people using conventional technologies.

This lecture begins with an overview of the importance of the approaches and techniques used to design ZETs for health and rehabilitation, including a discussion of the design principles that can be used in the development of effective ZETs. These principles are based on established design paradigms such as user-centred design and on the experiences of the authors that include: 1) understanding and incorporating real-world contexts; 2) complementing users' abilities; 3) the use of appropriate and intuitive interfaces; 4) encouraging user involvement and participation; 5) supporting the caregiver; 6) individualisation; 7) ensuring privacy and control; and 8) expandability and compatibility with other devices and technologies. The relevance of each of these principles to ZETs is discussed, including techniques that can be used to incorporate these principles and collect the necessary data to develop adaptive systems. This discussion is followed by a presentation of ZETs that have been developed and examples of how design principles have been applied to improve the

1. LECTURE OVERVIEW

safety and well-being of the people who rely on them. The lecture concludes with a summary of key limitations and future opportunities for ZETs.

CHAPTER 2

Introduction to Zero Effort Technologies

The scope and abilities of computer science and electronics are continuing to rapidly expand, resulting in the incorporation of technology into virtually all aspects of our lives. The purpose of technology is to enable people to do things they could not otherwise do, or to complete a task with greater efficiency, effectiveness, and safety—i.e., they increase people's abilities by providing assistance in completing tasks and activities. In order to be effective, technologies must somehow capture the context in which they are being used. This has traditionally been achieved through direct user input, with the person or people using the device providing explicit and specific input. The majority of technologies attempt to minimize user interactions and effort so that they place as few demands on the user as possible. Technology developers make an effort to optimally balance a device's applicability, customisability, and effectiveness with input requirements, which can often result in user burden and frustration, particularly if these inputs are required at specific times or if a missed input results in poor device performance. The ability of technologies to capture, analyse, and share data makes them a powerful tool in supporting people's health and well-being. However, it is especially important to consider the capabilities of users when developing technologies intended for people with impairments that may limit their abilities to access and operate the systems, such as people with cognitive disabilities. People with impairments are often unable to reliably initiate technology use and may not possess the skills, such as procedural memory, required to operate them.

2.1 WHAT IS A ZET?

Zero-effort technologies (ZETs) is a new class of technologies that employ techniques such as artificial intelligence and unobtrusive sensors to support the autonomous collection, analysis, and application of data about users and their context. The definitive aspect of ZETs is that they operate with minimal or no explicit feedback from the user, which translates into minimal or no learning or behaviour modification requirements for the users. In other words, ZETs are designed so that the people who use them do not have to change how they go about their daily lives and the ZETs will support them appropriately. As such, ZETs have tremendous potential to provide support to people with chronic health conditions with little or no effort on the part of the primary user or associated caregivers or clinicians.

Smart homes are a common example of ZETs that are being developed to support people's health and wellness. As illustrated in Figure 2.1, such an environment would be able to unobtrusively

4 2. INTRODUCTION TO ZERO EFFORT TECHNOLOGIES

monitor the actions of an occupant, learning about their preferences, abilities, changes in health, etc. As the occupant goes about his/her normal routine, the home will provide appropriate assistance

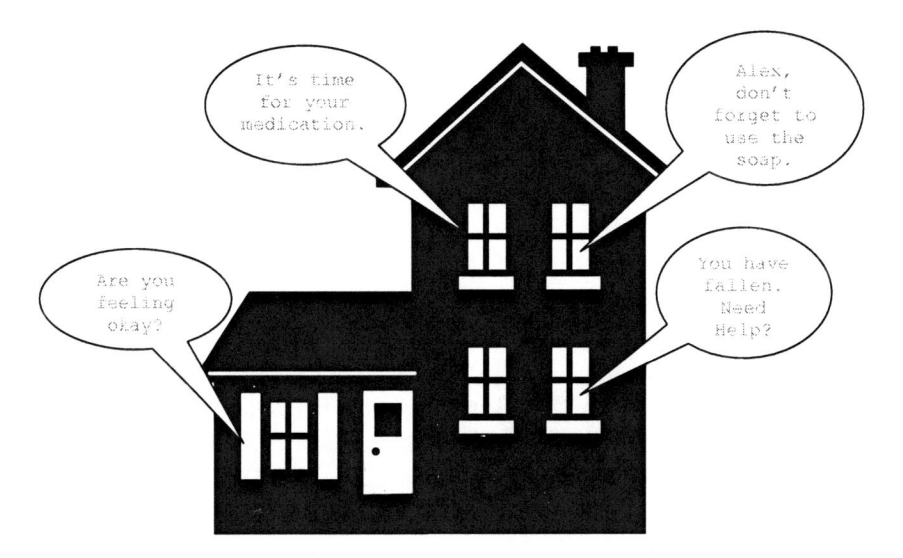

Figure 2.1: A typical example of a ZET is a smart home, that no matter the context or activity the occupant is trying to complete, the system provides appropriate assistance.

only as needed. This assistance may include detecting that it is time for the user to take his/her medication, and providing an appropriate prompt to do so. In this scenario, appropriate actions by the system may include detecting that the user is about to go out for a walk and determining whether he/she should be prompted to take the required medications before leaving. The house may also detect that the user, who has dementia, is attempting to complete a common self-care activity, such as handwashing, but has become confused on how to complete the activity. In response, the home provides a verbal reminder and ensures that the activity as been completed successfully. Finally, the system may have the ability to monitor the overall actions and movements of the occupant, learning about his/her daily living patterns, such as how often he/she uses the washroom or when he/she typically goes to bed. If changes in these usual patterns are detected, such as the person using the washroom twice as many times as per usual, the home can then automatically call for assistance and/or check in on the user. Through all of these different actions that the home system completes the key principle is that there is no effort required from the user to operate or interact with the various devices and components. The user lives his/her life as would typically be done, and the technology incorporates itself into the user's daily life. This is the main premise of ZETs.

For a technology to be zero-effort it does not necessarily mean that the user does not interact with the device. Rather, it means that interventions appropriately complement the different capabilities, expectations, and goals of the people using the device so that there is no *perceived* effort. For

2.1. WHAT IS A ZET? 5

example, take the previous example of a device built monitor a person's day-to-day routines in the home and detect when there is a deviation. For the person being monitored, the device would be zero-effort if he or she does not have to do anything for the device to operate; he or she would not have to activate the system, wear any markers or tags, set or change system parameters, or otherwise interact with the device for it to work. For the person's clinician, who would be interested in viewing trends in the person's health, the device could automatically generate suitable summaries, identify points that may be of interest to the clinician, and raise an alert if a potentially significant situation is detected. This data would be presented to the clinician in an intuitive format that could be easily manipulated, such as the ability for the clinician to drill-down or drill-up to gain a more holistic understanding of the person's health. Similarly, trends in health could be presented to the person who was being monitored and/or his or her family, enabling proactive health management. The data displayed to the person being monitored and their family would likely be in a simplified, easy to understand format compared to the data that would be presented to a clinician. Importantly, it would not be a requirement that the person being monitored and their family view or interact with the data if they did not wish to do so, rather it would be an option for users who wished to do so. Thus, such a device would be sensitive and accommodating to the variety of needs and abilities of the various users and stakeholders, enabling effortless access to the items and functions relevant to his or her interests and abilities.

In order to implement many of the ideals of ZETs various upcoming areas from computer science are required that can help provide the intelligent, flexibility, and comprehensiveness needed by this new class of technologies. A primary field of interest to the development of ZETs is *pervasive computing*. The words pervasive means "existing everywhere," hence pervasive computing is the incorporation of microprocessors and sensors in everyday objects and environments so they can seamlessly and efficiently capture and communicate information. Pervasive computing aims to create applications where all the devices that are involved are completely connected and constantly available, enabling direct and customised responses to users and environments with a greatly reduced need for explicit human guidance. Pervasive computing relies on the convergence of wireless technologies, advanced electronics, and networks, such as intranets and the Internet. When pervasive computing products are connected to the Internet, the data they generate can easily be made available in any place and at any time (e.g., health data collected about a patient can be easily accessed by the user's family physician). Security measures are put in place to protect users' privacy and ensure that only intended recipients have access to the specific data they have been granted access to. The principles surrounding pervasive computing are discussed in detail in the following section.

One of the key concepts that the field of pervasive computing, and hence ZETs, is based on is *context-aware computing*. Context can be broadly defined as any information that helps to define the needs, preferences, abilities, and the circumstances that may form the setting in which a person may participate in a particular activity. Contextual factors, as will be explained in more detail later in this lecture, can be defined as personal (e.g., age, gender, type of disability) and as environmental (e.g., type of environment, lighting conditions, other people sharing the space) [1]. Context aware computing attempts to collect all of the data required for the developed system to provide a more customized approach in its operation [2]. This premise is critically important in the application of pervasive computing as it is these data that allows ZETs to have the adaptability and intelligence required to reduce the perceived effort of operation on their users. This lecture will not provide any depth on this particular topic, as this concept is embedded in the various principles of pervasive computing and artificial intelligence (as will be covered further in this lecture). For more details on this field of work and relevant research that has been completed, the reader is referred to more in-depth literature, such as [3–6].

Finally, in order to implement many of the principles of pervasive computing and context-awareness, concepts from *artificial intelligence* (AI) are a key feature of ZETs. AI techniques can be used to manipulate and interpret incoming data, making it possible for ZETs to identify and respond to situations or trends of interest in an appropriate fashion. As such, ZETs are able to perform autonomous data manipulation, which allows the targeted and customisable presentation of data in formats that are tailored to the interests of different stakeholders, such as clinicians, professional and informal caregivers, and, importantly, the person being assisted.

2.2 OVERVIEW OF PERVASIVE COMPUTING

Pervasive computing is an effort to make information-centric tasks simple, mobile, and secure [7]. Pervasive computing devices are not personal computers, but are either mobile or embedded in almost any type of object imaginable, including cars, tools, appliances, clothing and various consumer goods—all communicating through interconnected networks. Research in this field has primarily been aimed at improving the efficiency of current and new computing applications by making them available in more places, more often, and with more convenience for users. The ability to provide immense flexibility while simultaneously reducing user demands has resulted in a relatively quick uptake and implementation of pervasive computing applications, including ZETs for supporting health, rehabilitation, and well-being.

While application in healthcare is a relatively new area of research in pervasive computing, this concept has already been adopted in other areas. One recent trend relates to technologies that support energy management and specifically 'smart grid' systems [8], which is presented here to illustrate how the principles of pervasive computing may apply in practice. The IEEE's conceptual model [9] depicts the multiple and bi-directional energy and information channels between stakeholders, hinting at the flexibility and interrelated nature of this system (see Figure 2.2). This example will be used in the proceeding sub-sections to illustrate various concepts related to pervasive computing, primarily the four principles used in this field.

2.2.1 PERVASIVE COMPUTING PRINCIPLES

Pervasive computing is based on four fundamental paradigms: 1) decentralization; 2) diversification; 3) connectivity; and 4) simplicity [10].

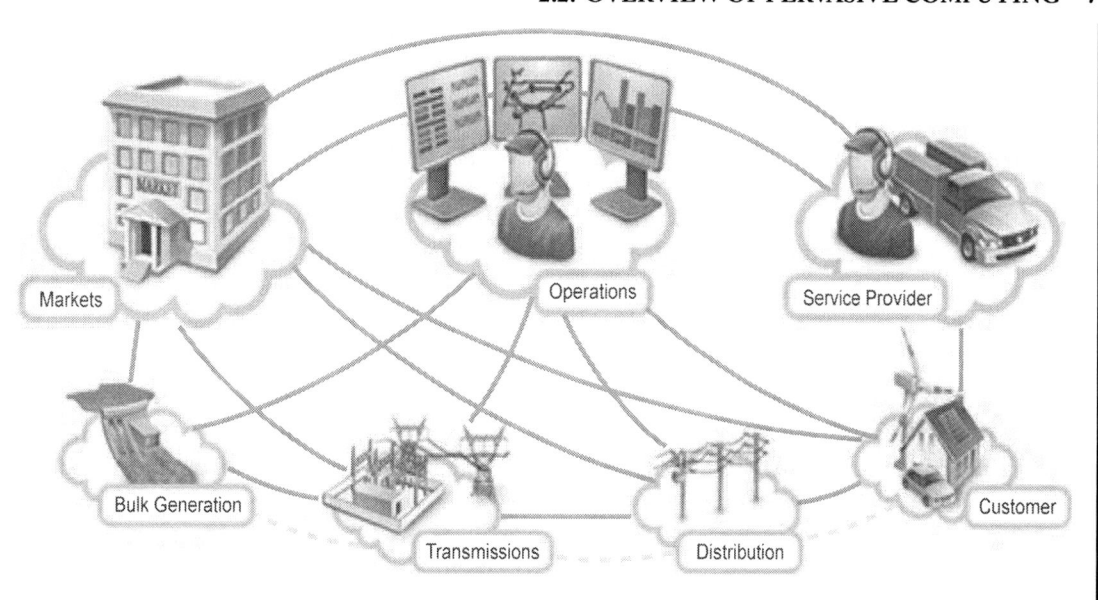

Figure 2.2: A specific example of the use of pervasive computing outside of the healthcare domain. The IEEE's conceptual model of 'smart grids' [9], involving technologies that are intended to be distributed, diverse, interconnected and, for the customer, simple to use.

The first principle of pervasive computing is *decentralization*. Typically, computing systems have been based on a centralized component, such as a computer server, which manages and runs all of the required computer processes. In contrast to this traditional approach, decentralization is when a system uses many devices that each performs a specialized task or tasks. In this way, pervasive computing distributes a system's responsibilities between a variety of small devices or sub-systems, each of which take over specific tasks and functionality [10]. As each sub-system can perform some measure of independent data collection and analysis, decentralization enables large amounts of data to be captured as each sub-system is able to perform some measure of pre-processing on the data it captures. This reduces or eliminates hardware bottlenecks and increases the transfer rate of data between sub-systems, as pre-processing allows filtering and logic operations to be applied to data pre-transmission as well as enabling techniques such as event-driven communication to be exploited. Moreover, decentralization can increase a system's robustness as it may still be able to operate effectively even if one or more sub-systems fail.

This notion of decentralization is already well entrenched within smart grid designs. Conventional power systems typically involve a large power plant that distributes energy downstream to end-users who possess no real-time information on rates or usage. Modernization of power technology, however, may significantly shift this paradigm [11]. Not only are multiple sources of energy, including renewable energies, now being utilized, but applications that offer customers real-time information with which to make energy choices are under development [12], as are opt-in plans for pervasive, non-intrusive circuitry to learn and control appliance use [13]. Thus, home area networks may be coordinated with ubiquitous sensor networks and operations-level networks to monitor, analyze, control, and troubleshoot power delivery [9].

The second principle, *diversification*, builds upon the notion of decentralization. In typical computing applications, a system performs all necessary applications on a "universal" computer. Diversification, on the other hand, is the ability to employ several different types of devices and computing units for each sub-system, where these devices may be different "classes" of technologies, each with its own unique capabilities, inputs, and outputs. For example, a pervasive computing system can employ smart phones, laptops, and various sensors where all of these devices are able to communicate with each other and the overall system (using common communication protocols as will be described). Diversity in the devices that can be used is important because as individual sub-systems are intended for a specific situation or environment, they can be optimized for their particular context or contexts [10]. A key aspect to ensuring that diversified systems operate effectively and efficiently is to manage the resulting diversity of data that often accompanies the use of multiple different types of devices. Data management can be particularly challenging when integrating data from different user interfaces and data input mechanisms, which can include autonomously, semi-autonomously, and manually input data captured using different computing platforms and operating systems. Interoperability between sub-systems is accomplished through the use of standards and protocols that enable different devices to perform common features and functions, which are described in more detail later in the lecture.

In the case of smart grids, not only are different forms of energy increasingly being utilized, but also different kinds of information processing devices: home area networks are populated with smart appliances and smart meters, while non-intrusive load control circuitry functions, in part, via networks of sensors that feed into artificially intelligent algorithms [13]. These various kinds of devices meet specific requirements within the broader system, thereby diversifying the grid.

The third principle, *connectivity*, attempts to resolve issues that may arise from the use of many different devices that have different user interfaces, control mechanisms, and communication protocols. While the premise of pervasive computing is to allow for the decentralization and diversity in the devices and algorithms that are implemented, there still needs to be uniformity in how these devices communicate. This is true not only for the sub-systems within a single pervasive computing system, but for communication between these systems as well. For example, interoperability requires that the same communication protocols are used by pervasive computing devices and services to enable data transfer between systems, such as data sharing between home monitoring devices and a central data repository. As pervasive systems become more widely applied, connectivity standards continue to be developed and adopted, such as WAP, UMTS, Bluetooth, or IrDA [10], and are described in more detail later in this lecture.

This principle of connectivity applies to smart grids also because although energy networks function independently, they, too, must be capable of communicating seamlessly. To meet this requirement, 'Smart grid interoperability standards' [14] have been catalogued by the National Institute of Science and Technology (NIST). These standards render communication within the broader power system possible.

The final principle, *simplicity*, is perhaps the most important principle of pervasive computing for the development of ZETs aimed at supporting healthcare and rehabilitation. Pervasive computing has a heavy focus on issues related to human-computer interaction (HCI). One way ZETs ensure there is no or almost no learning curve is by ensuring systems are so intuitive that people can use them as easily as common everyday products [7, 15]. Some interfaces are more conventional, such as energy management applications that operate on home computers to provide real-time rate information, so customers can monitor and control appliance use [12]. However, as many pervasive computing devices are embedded into an environment or are small mobile devices, they cannot necessarily support the same kinds of input devices (e.g., keyboard, mouse) that are used with traditional platforms, such as a personal computer. The novel platforms used in pervasive computing devices have driven the development of new approaches and techniques that allow users to easily interface and interact with devices in non-traditional ways. For example, control of a device using speech represents a user interface that may be more intuitive for some user types. The principle of simplicity is also critical when developing technologies for people with disabilities or older adults. These user groups tend to have decreased capacities as a result of physical, cognitive, or sensory impairments and thus greatly benefit when they are able to interact with technologies in a way that is simple, intuitive, and requires no learning.

2.2.2 ELEMENTS OF PERVASIVE COMPUTING SYSTEMS

For any pervasive computing system to be effective, there needs to be three different components developed and taken into consideration: 1) the devices that run developed applications; 2) the protocols and standards that allow devices and applications to communicate; and 3) the applications and services provided by pervasive computing [15].

Devices

There is a wide range of different *devices* that can be part of a pervasive computing system. Any device that is considered to be useful to the system can be employed and can range from devices, such as smart phones, to more "traditional" computing devices such as desktop computers and data servers. The latter devices often provide behind the scenes support for the mobile components of a pervasive application and require other devices such as network routers and modems, mobile phone towers, and wireless access points to be included in the system [15]. With respect to the previous smart grid example, devices that are being used in that domain include personal computers located within the homes of customers, sensors that detect environmental conditions within the home, and common appliances such as thermostats, furnaces, and air conditioners.

Many advanced pervasive computing systems, including a number of applications related to healthcare and rehabilitation, rely heavily on sensors that can monitor various aspects of an environment. Examples of sensors include motion detectors, radio-frequency identification (RFID) devices, video cameras, and motion capture systems. Using data from these sensors, systems can act upon the environment and/or a user through the use of another set of devices, known as actuators. Some examples of actuators are switches that can autonomously turn off a stove or the lights, or can send an alert to a person's mobile device. A more detailed discussion of sensors and actuators is presented in Section 2.3.1.

Standards and Protocols
In order to support the principle of diversity in the types of devices and applications that can be used, *standards and protocols* are essential to allow different systems to share information. At the hardware level, standards and protocols are needed to specify how devices should collect and output data to ensure that all other devices can understand the messages and data the device transmits or needs to receive [15]. In addition, protocols are used to define how to package information, address messages to different recipients, to ensure messages or data have arrived at their intended destinations, and to ensure that data is not lost or compromised during transmission. At both the hardware and software levels, protocols and standards are also needed to ensure adequate security is built into a system. This includes ensuring that a user or a device has permission to access a resource and preventing non-authorized users and systems from "listening" to messages [15]. Issues regarding security in pervasive computing and ZETs are presented later in this lecture.

There have been many different standards and protocols developed at both the hardware and software levels. Two of the most relevant and widely used hardware standards include UPnP (Universal plug and play) and the Tivoli device management system [10, 15]. Using these protocols, device manufacturers can describe the kinds of information that their hardware produces and accepts. By clearly providing this information, different devices can be readily integrated into heterogeneous networks. With these protocols in place all a user typically has to do is add a new device to an existing network and the system automatically identifies the device and downloads the necessary drivers and applications. This type of automatic, "plug and play" network configuration is at the heart of the pervasive computing paradigm, as one goal of pervasive computing is for devices to be seamlessly integrated into existing systems, whenever and wherever they are needed [15]. As previously described, NIST has developed the 'Smart grid interoperability standards' [14] for smart power grid systems.

The ability for different devices to automatically and effortlessly be integrated into an existing architecture addresses a key area in the development of ZETs, which is to enable compatibility between different devices and systems. For example, the issue of cross compatibility is becoming very important in new smart home systems that are being developed to help people with disabilities complete a variety of tasks and activities of daily living. Currently, many of the available technologies are proprietary, stand alone systems that require a considerable effort from software developers before they are able to talk with each other. If an UPnP protocol was implemented during their development, each of the smart home devices would be able to automatically pass data back and forth to other smart home systems as soon as it was installed.

Closely tied to hardware-based protocols and standards are those related to communication networks. Network protocols have existed for many years with the most common and well recognised being the TCP/IP (Transmission Control Protocol/Internet Protocol) [15]. TCP/IP is built into many operating systems (e.g., Windows, Linux, Mac-OS) and is the protocol used by the Internet. This protocol is one way of specifying the addresses of different devices in a network and ensuring that messages are correctly sent from one device to another across a network. Other protocols have been built on top of TCP/IP, such as HTTP (Hypertext Transfer Protocol), which is a communication protocol for transferring data on the World Wide Web. HTTP is a server-client based protocol where one system, called the client (e.g., a web browser), makes a request to another system, called the server (e.g., a web server), for particular data (e.g., files) [15]. The server interprets the client's request, and if the request is considered to be genuine, passes the relevant data back to the client.

The dramatic increase in the use of mobile devices, such as smart phones, has resulted in large and rapid increases in the development of protocols and standards related to these pervasive computing devices. This includes protocols for cellular telephone communication (e.g., GSM, TDMA, CDMA, GPRS, and SMS), Bluetooth (which is a standard that supports communication devices that use a particular type of small, inexpensive radio chip), and Wireless Application Protocol (WAP; which is similar to HTTP but specifically for use with mobile platforms) [15].

Application Services

The primary objective of pervasive computing is to develop applications and services that can be used effectively in a variety of contexts. The purpose of developing devices, standards and protocols is to provide the infrastructure that is needed by these applications [15]. Pervasive computing covers a wide range of applications from communication (including email, telephones, text messaging, and video conferencing) to data management and analysis, such as database access and file transfer. For example, as part of the new smart power grid systems, many consumer hydro and power providers have developed "easy-to-use" web-based portals that consumers can log into and view their current power consumptions, and ways of further reducing their power usage and costs. As pervasive computing infrastructure continues to mature, more sophisticated applications and services will continue to emerge. This has been the case for healthcare applications, where new pervasive computing systems are being developed and deployed to help in the care of patients in hospitals, clinics, and within the home. Pervasive computing in healthcare has included applications and services aimed at reducing the cost of providing healthcare, increasing the quality of care provided to patients, providing peace of mind and assistance to family caregivers, and assisting in the management of chronic conditions. Examples of such systems related to healthcare and rehabilitation is provided in Chapter 5 of this lecture.

2. INTRODUCTION TO ZERO EFFORT TECHNOLOGIES

Security and Privacy in Pervasive Computing

The premise of pervasive computing and its principles makes systems possible targets to security threats. Making information available to users in more places and at more times requires increased collection and transmission of data, which provides additional opportunities to those who wish to steal or corrupt information [10, 15]. Intimately related to security is the notion of privacy, which is an assurance that a piece of information is only accessed by specified users or devices [10, 15]. Pervasive computing systems can be vulnerable to privacy threats as information and data typically need to be transmitted through media that is shared by other people, such as the Internet. As a result, trade-offs exist between security, privacy, convenience, and cost that need to be incorporated into the design of any pervasive computing system. For example, typing in passwords or waiting for authorization to use resources can be a hassle, but one that is reasonable and acceptable for applications that contain sensitive data.

As more devices and applications are connected to each other, this need for multiple authorizations to occur increases, and as such, the aforementioned tradeoffs become even more important. These considerations can be particularly challenging to implement in healthcare technologies as overburdened healthcare workers and caregivers do not have the time to be continuously authenticating themselves, and users who have a disability may not have the capacities required to do so. However, no user will, or should, accept a system where personal details regarding themselves and the people they care for are vulnerable to security risks. As such, it is not an option to consider security in these systems as an after-thought in the design process; security and privacy need to be incorporated at all stages in the design process of any ZET. This goal can be achieved through a framework known as *Privacy By Design*, which was developed by the Information Privacy Commission of Ontario [16]. Details of the privacy by design framework and its relevance to ZETs and other assistive technologies are presented in Section 3.1.3 of this lecture.

2.3 OVERVIEW OF AI PRINCIPLES

The diverse characteristics of the potential users of ZETs (e.g., people with disabilities and their families) make it that one solution cannot fit all users. A user-centred design approach (which is discussed later in this lecture) needs to be used to ensure that ZETs are flexible and are able to meet the various needs of each individual user as much as possible. However, manually applying this approach can be extremely costly, very time consuming, and is difficult to support on an ongoing basis. Furthermore, any technology developed needs to also be operated by the primary user's caregivers, family members, and support group—i.e., it needs to be universally designed to take into account a wide variety of abilities, needs, and preferences (as will be discussed later in this lecture). In response, there has been an increase in the number of projects in the field of assistive technology that are applying sophisticated paradigms and approaches, such as artificial intelligence (AI), to reduce, simplify, or negate explicit user interactions. AI allows for technologies to be developed that can autonomously sense, learn, and adapt to individual users, lending itself well to tasks that involve learning and decision-making. AI helps researchers to design ZETs that are able to operate within

2.3. OVERVIEW OF AI PRINCIPLES 13

a user-centred design framework by enabling the device to autonomously customise support to the individual needs of each user. *Sensing* and *machine learning* are two AI techniques that are especially useful in achieving autonomous operation, customisability, and usability in ZETs, therefore the remainder of this section presents an overview of the application of sensing and machine learning to the development of ZETs.

2.3.1 COMMONLY USED SENSING TECHNIQUES

A critical feature of any ZET is its ability to sense the environment to determine what a user is trying to do, namely, how he or she is interacting with his or her environment. There is no definitive type of sensor for ZETs, rather the sensor or sensor network that is used depends on the purpose, design criteria, and specific application of the ZET. Moreover, in theory, a ZET can be expanded to include other sensors, or even other ZETs or systems, as the particular implementation requires.

Sensors can be classified according to different criteria, such as whether they are active or passive (i.e., whether they actively transmit data or not), worn on the person or installed within the environment, and are capable of wired or wireless communication. Within these broad categories there are sensor types that are more commonly used in the development of ZETs, which are: 1) sensors that are embedded into an environment; 2) portable or wearable sensors; and 3) vision-based sensors (i.e., cameras and computer vision). A high-level summary of these different types of sensors is presented below. Interested readers can refer to a recent survey article for details and further references on embedded or portable sensors, such as Chen (2011) [17], and to Szeliski (2010) [18] or Bradski (2008) [19] for computer vision.

It is important to keep in mind that most sensors require power and that all sensors need to communicate over a network in some way to transmit data. Appropriate cables must be run for wired sensors and the user must change batteries or otherwise charge wireless sensors. Sensors also range in cost, which usually reflects their complexity and accuracy. Developers need to carefully consider these aspects to ensure that the sensors that are incorporated into a ZET's infrastructure are appropriate for the population, environment, and activity that are being monitored.

Embedded Sensors

This class of sensors consists of a wide variety of sensors that are usually low cost, commercially available, and are often meant to measure a single factor or signal. One of the most commonly used environmental sensors in ZETs is a motion detector that simply detects the presence of motion within a specific room. There are several versions of this type of sensor, including motion sensors that use optical, acoustical, or infrared changes in the field of view to detect motion. Motion sensors can also include occupancy sensors, which integrate a timing device to measure how long a person may be within or absent from the area being monitored by the sensor.

Motion sensors are just one example of an environmental sensor. Other commonly used environmental sensors include devices that can measure specific events, such as mechanical devices that measure water usage, thermostats that measure environmental temperature and humidity, and microswitches that can detect if a person is lying on a bed, sitting on a chair, or has opened a door. Importantly, most sensors are only able to measure one or two aspects of an environment, usually monitor a limited area, and transmit minimal, often binary, information. For example, microswitches can only detect whether the particular door or cupboard they are attached to is open or closed. They cannot give information about how far a door is open (i.e., whether a door is fully open or open just a crack) or give information about whether someone walked through the door (as opposed to just opening it) or is interacting with items in a cupboard. Additionally, a sensor must be installed for each area or item that the ZET needs to monitor, such as a microswitch for each door of interest.

Portable or Wearable Sensors
Portable or wearable sensors are designed to attach to a person or object and collect and/or transmit data without being physically connected to a network. As they are intended to be mobile and as unobtrusive as possible, the majority of portable sensors have small form factors and are lightweight. There is a wide range of portable sensors available, including accelerometers, gyroscopes, thermisters, and heart rate monitors. As with embedded sensors, the number and types of portable sensors used in a ZET is dependent on the specific application and more than one type of sensor may be used.

Radiofrequency-based sensors are an example of a portable sensor that has achieved widespread use and is becoming increasingly prevalent in ZETs. This is because of the relatively low cost and robust performance of these sensors. A common type of radiofrequency-based sensor is Radio Frequency Identification (RFID), which consists of 'readers' and 'tags'. Readers are usually installed at fixed points in an environment and are able to sense the presence of the tags, which are worn by a person or placed on objects of interest. A communication protocol allows the reader to detect when a tag is nearby and to identify which tag it is sensing. RFID readers require power and can be hooked into a communication network such as an intranet or the Internet. RFID tags can be passive, active, or battery-assisted passive (BAP). A passive tag generally only contains the identification number of the tag and the information contained on the tag usually cannot be altered once the tag has been assembled. In a passive RFID system, the reader periodically sends out a signal, and if the passive tag is within range, the reader can detect the presence of the tag and can identify which tag it is detecting. Using powered supplied by the reader, the coiled antennae in the tag then generates a magnetic field from which power is drawn in order to send information from the tag back to the reader, such as the tag's unique ID. Passive tags must be within a few meters of a reader to be detected. One example of the use of RFIDs is in security badges, which a user must swipe across a reader, and if the tag's ID has been registered, the reader will unlock the door. An active tag uses a battery to power the tag and is able to collect and actively transmit and receive limited amounts of data stored in its memory back to a reader. These data include the identification number assigned to the tag, but can also contain more descriptive information, such as the last known location of the tag. Similar to a beacon, active systems can be used for real-time locating by actively emitting a signal to a reader at pre-set intervals. Active tags can also be 'pinged' by a reader, meaning that they transmit data to a reader only upon receiving a signal from a reader to do so. Implementing this pinging technique can greatly reduce a tag's power consumption (as data transmission is relatively power intensive) and can increase network security as the tag is not continuously transmitting data. Active tags typically have transmission ranges of up to 300 feet, although this range can be less if obstructions or radio frequency noise are present. A BAP tag incorporates other sensors such as temperature, humidity, and illumination. As such, it can collect, store, and transmit much greater amounts of data, however, this requires a larger, often external battery, which is heavier and can require more frequent recharging. The reader is referred to Want (2006) [20] for a more in-depth discussion of RFID sensors and technologies.

While the particulars may be different, many portable or wearable sensors operate in a similar fashion to RFID systems. Some sensors are capable of large and rapid capture and transmission of data, others are more passive and simple in nature. However, enhanced capabilities usually have greater power needs, resulting in heavier batteries and devices that require recharging more often. Therefore, a ZET developer strives for the optimal balance between a device's data capture and transmission capabilities and the device's power requirements.

Vision-Based Sensors
The use of vision-based sensors in ZETS, such as web cameras, is becoming increasingly popular as a result of decreasing hardware costs, vast improvements in image processing algorithms with respect to computational costs and robustness, and the recognition that the rich data set that can be collected can be used for a variety of applications. With respect to the latter point, vision-based sensors can not only collect data that other sensor types cannot, but can reduce the number of sensors required to monitor an activity or environment.

Computer vision is when a computer is used to apply various image/video processing techniques to extract information from an image or series of images (video) that is then used for another type of application. Image processing techniques include object recognition, activity recognition, motion analysis, scene reconstruction, and image restoration. In *object/activity recognition*, an image is analysed to see if it contains a specific object, feature, or activity of interest. This is achieved by the system learning what the object or activity looks like based on training data that contains various features and poses that enable the system to recognise the object or activity when the system sees it. This can be a quite challenging endeavour. For example, if a system using computer vision needs to know when a person has sat in a chair, it must be able to recognise what a chair looks like, what a person looks like, and when the person is sitting in the chair. When considering the chair alone, the system must be able to recognise many styles of chairs and that a chair can look very different from different angles (i.e., if the chair is moved or rotated) and in different lighting conditions. *Motion analysis* tracks a target object, such as a person, and is typically used in ZETs to determine what a person is doing. This is achieved by algorithms that analyse sequential video frames and compare the object of interest from one frame to the next to determine if the object is moving and, if so, in what direction and by how much. A key aspect of motion analysis is the ability of the system to differentiate the object being tracked from the background and other (irrelevant) features in the environment. Introductory texts on computer vision include Szeliski (2010) [18], Shapiro & Stockman (2001) [21], and Forsyth and Ponce (2002) [22]. Duda and Hart (2000) [23] and Bishop (2006) [24] also include many computer vision applications of machine learning. The most well-known practical introduction to computer vision is provided by the openCV toolkit, an open-source set of libraries for a wide variety of computer vision tasks [19].

2.3.2 COMMONLY USED MACHINE LEARNING APPROACHES

Machine learning (ML) is an area of AI concerned with the study and creation of computer algorithms that improve automatically through exposure to data. This area of AI is extremely important in the development and usability of ZETs as even users from the same population can be quite different and a person's habits can change drastically over time. However, so far there has not been much literature on this area within the context of ZETs and other technologies for healthcare and rehabilitation, as these fields and applications are relatively new. As such, a more detailed presentation of ML and its applicability to ZETs will be provided in this section.

There are a variety of different ML techniques that have been developed and each has its strengths and weaknesses, causing different ML algorithms to be better suited to different types of problems. In all cases, the basic idea is for the system to learn a function that maps between some inputs (e.g., sensor readings in a smart home or database query results) and some outputs (e.g., identifying a human behaviour or selecting an action for a system to take). For example, if the system detects that a flow meter is running and that the level of water in a sink is very high (inputs) it means that it should shut the water off before the sink overflows (output).

ML is often achieved using a data set that represents the problem of interest. After learning is complete, the system is evaluated on a separate set of test examples, which can be a portion of the data set that was not shown to the system in the training data or a sample of similar data from other scenarios. The metric for success is the performance of the system when interpreting and reacting to the test examples; a ML algorithm is considered to be successful if it is able to map what it learned with the training data to perform successfully on the test data. A ML algorithm can perform very well on the training data, but if it has created a mapping that is too specific to the training data, it will not be able to recognise situations of interest in other contexts and will fail when it encounters other test or real-world data. This phenomenon of performing well with training data but failing in other contexts is called "overfitting".

Machine learning algorithms can be grouped into three categories that describe how the learning is accomplished: 1) supervised learning; 2) unsupervised learning; and 3) reinforcement learning. There are a growing number of different ML techniques in each of these three learning categories, and a review of ZET literature shows that methods from all three categories are being used in the development of new technologies. These methods are briefly discussed in the remainder of this section. The particular machine learning techniques and methods are highly dependant on the nature of the problem that is being modelled as well as other parameters, such as how much training data is available and how well this data represents the intended real-world application.

2.3. OVERVIEW OF AI PRINCIPLES 17

Therefore, software developers must work closely with other members of the research team, such as engineers and end-users, to ensure that the problem is well defined and an appropriate machine learning technique applied.

The remainder of this subsection provides an overview of these three categories and examples of specific ML algorithms for each. Details on the ML concepts introduced in this section can be found in texts on machine learning [24–27] and artificial intelligence [28], [29].

Russell and Norvig (1995) [29] provides a very detailed overall introduction to the field of Artificial Intelligence and Machine Learning. Poole and Mackworth (2010) [28] approach AI from a logical perspective, presenting a simple and approachable introduction to the field. Bishop (2006) [24] and MacKay (2003) [25] provide more detailed insights into machine learning in particular. MacKay (2003) [25] in particular investigates the Bayesian learning paradigm in great detail. Reinforcement learning is covered by Sutton (1998) [27]. Duda, Hart and Stork (2002) [23] give an excellent introduction to pattern analysis and machine learning, including aspects of computer vision. WEKA (www.cs.waikato.ac.nz/ml/weka) is a suite of Machine Learning tools with open-source implementations provided online, including documentation of the various approaches. WEKA is usually used as a starting point for the application of ML and/or AI techniques. AISpace is a suite of Java Applets that demonstrate a variety of ML/AI techniques and can be used for learning/training purposes (www.aispace.org).

Supervised Learning
Supervised learning is one of the most common and well known ML approaches. In supervised learning, the data set that will be used to develop an algorithm (or model) is first labelled by an expert (usually a human). The algorithm is then presented with the training data, which consist of examples that include both the inputs and optimal corresponding outputs. For example, for a system that was being developed to use computer vision to recognise when someone was sitting in a chair, the training data set might consist of a number of videos filmed from different angles of people getting into and out of different types of chairs. For each video, a human expert would identify and label objects and situations of interest; in this example, the chair, the person, and whether the person was sitting in the chair or not. From these data, the algorithm can use the labelled data to learn relationships between objects and situations of interest so that it is able to identify and map, or classify, new inputs to appropriate outputs.

Typically, data for a supervised learning approach take the form of a number of inputs that can be discrete (taking on one of a set of values) or real-valued (taking on any real number), and an output (target). For example, in a ZET application, inputs may be the values of a number of sensors in an older adult's home, while the target attribute (output) may be a category of human activity. Inputs can represent a discrete (e.g., a switch that is on or off) or continuous (e.g., a temperature) condition of the world. Output is typically discrete (e.g., an activity is being performed or not), partially because this is generally simpler to model, but the variable can be continuous when warranted by the application, such as when a ZET is using outputs that are not directly observable (e.g., estimating a person's risk of falling).

The most well-used supervised learning technique for a model that uses discrete-valued target attributes is a *decision tree* [29, 30]. With a decision tree, input attributes are used to divide the data into sets, which are used to predict the target attribute with greater accuracy. *A decision tree* consists of a set of nodes arranged in a tree structure, each node being associated with a *test* of a set of input attributes (usually only one). The possible results of the test are represented as *branches* emanating from the node, leading to other, similar nodes or to *leaves* of the tree, each of which represents a target attribute value. Classification of a data sample proceeds from the root of the tree by applying a test at a node, and then following the branch that corresponds to the output of the test. This process is repeated until a leaf is reached, at which point the predicted target attribute is read off. A decision tree can be learned using a simple *greedy approach*. In the greedy approach, each input attribute is evaluated by its ability to divide the input data into sets that have similar output attribute values. The input attribute and test that performs best is then chosen as the root node. This process is repeated recursively for each test result and associated training data. The choices of attributes, how to split data based on those attributes, when to choose to stop splitting data, and when to create new branches are settings that will bias the final decision tree results. Therefore, carefully assigning and assessing these settings is key to learning an effective decision tree (i.e., one that generalises and is not overfitted). The standard text on decision tree learning is described in [30].

Another very popular supervised learning approach is the *neural network*. The neural network was one of the first forms of AI to emerge and attempts to emulate human intelligence on a machine by replicating the neuron-based learning that occurs in humans. In a neural network, each input attribute is assigned to an input node in a network of neuron-like processing units. Each artificial neuron takes values from a set of input nodes and compares a weighted sum of these values to a threshold, firing an output *pulse* if the threshold is crossed. A second layer of neurons then combines the outputs from the first layer in a similar way. The outputs of the second layer are predictors of the target attribute. The neural network is trained by repeated presentations of inputs, which results in a series of outputs. A simple update rule is used at each node to compare the outputs and bring the predictions closer to the true outputs. While this technique can be robust and versatile, training a neural network is often time consuming and may not be generalisable to other applications of interest. Chapter 5 of Bishop (2006) [24] contains a good overview of neural network training algorithms.

Unsupervised Learning

In many situations, it is difficult or undesirable to assign output labels to a set of training data. For example, a ZET could be used to autonomously detect changes in a person's daily routines. However, what constitutes a normal routine is drastically different from person to person; therefore, the ZET must first model (or learn) each individual's normal routines. After the normal routines are captured, new data can be compared to this normality model to see if there are any deviations and, if so, what

2.3. OVERVIEW OF AI PRINCIPLES 19

the deviations are. In applications such as these, it is not desirable or feasible to assign categories to a training set, but rather is important to learn the unique types of patterns are normally present in each particular deployment [31]. Unsupervised learning tackles problems such as these.

The most common unsupervised approaches are statistical in nature, where a statistical model is hypothesised and its parameters are learned by a computer from a set of data. The simplest example is the mixture model, where a probability distribution is defined over the input attributes given a set of (unknown but of fixed size) labels. These labels then constitute the target (output) attributes. An algorithm such as the expectation-maximization (EM) algorithm can then be used to learn the parameters of this probability distribution such that the likelihood of the data given the parameters is maximized. Mixture models can handle multi-dimensional, mixed continuous and discrete inputs and can learn output attributes with many values [24]. A generalisation is to learn parameters such that the probability of the parameters is maximized given the data (Bayesian learning). In this case, a prior probability distribution over the parameters is necessary to encode all prior information that is available about the model. In this case, one usually assumes that the *number* of parameters is known beforehand (e.g., the number of target output labels we expect to see). A further generalisation removes this restriction, and allows the model to also learn the *number* of output values or labels by placing a prior distribution over this number. The resulting model will be able to learn both the values of the parameters and the number (and type) of parameters. These methods are known as hierarchical Bayesian learning or nonparametric Bayesian learning methods. Such methods have been used recently in many text categorisation and machine translation problems [32] and have started to be applied to ZETs.

Unsupervised learning can be seen as a form of clustering, in which a computer searches for patterns in the data. The *clustering objective* is to create the optimum number and size of subsets of input data such that the data within each subset are all very similar (small intra-class distance) and all the data in different subsets are very dissimilar (large inter-class distance). Many clustering approaches exist, the simplest of which is based on computing the ordered eigenvectors of the input data (also known as principal components analysis; PCA). The principal (first) eigenvector is a vector in the high-dimensional space of input attributes along which the data are the most variable (or dissimilar). Splitting the input data into two sets at the mid-point of this vector is often an effective method for finding sets that satisfy the clustering goal. A recursive application of this method is referred to as *vector quantization*. See Chapter 12 in Bishop (2006) [24], or Chapter 10 in Duda and Hart (2002) [23] for more details.

Neural networks can be used for clustering. The self-organising map (SOM) is a classic example of a neural network with an unsupervised training rule [33]. In a similar fashion to the supervised case, SOMs are trained by slowly adjusting the weights of each neuron. However, the adjustments cannot be made to bring the predictions in line with the true outputs (as the learning is unsupervised), therefore some other measures of success must be used. Maximizing the entropy of the target labels given the inputs is one approach that attempts to satisfy an objective similar to the one defined above for clustering. See Chapter 5 of Bishop (2006) [24] for more details.

Bayesian networks (BNs) provide a framework for modelling uncertainty that can be used for both supervised and unsupervised learning. Many of the techniques we have been discussing under these headings can be formulated as BNs, and powerful learning techniques exist to adapt these models to data. See Koller (2009) [34] for details.

Reinforcement Learning
In reinforcement learning (RL) [27], an agent (i.e., something that perceives and acts) explores the environment and receives a reward upon achieving a goal. Rewards can be positive or negative to encourage the agent to take actions that will be the most likely to result in desirable states and dissuade actions that will likely result in undesirable states. RL can be seen as a form of supervised learning in which the output (target) labels are the reward values. The difficulty with RL is that the reward is often delayed, namely rewards may only be attainable in states that are not immediately achievable therefore the agent must take several actions before gaining a positive reward, possibly risking gaining negative rewards (i.e., a negative value of reward or "punishment" associated with undesirable states) in the process. For example, a personal assistant robot may only learn that it has done a good job at the end of the day when its performance is evaluated. It will not know which specific actions led to that reward signal. The agent therefore needs to learn how to act so that, in the long run, it achieves the maximum cumulative reward. The function that tells an agent what to do in any situation is known as a *policy* [27].

There are two major types of RL algorithms: model-based and model-free. In a model-based approach, the agent assumes some parameterized model of the dynamics of the environment (and of its actions in it) and of the rewards. The agent then gathers evidence (observations) about these parameters while acting in the world. Once the model has been learned, a policy can be computed that optimises the reward function. The advantages of a model-based approach are that it is easily interpretable and prior knowledge about the domain is relatively easy to incorporate. Model-free approaches, on the other hand, do not assume a model, rather the agent must attempt to learn the policy directly from the data. The advantage of model-free approaches is that there is less bias imposed on the structure of the environment and more complex dynamics can be learned given enough data. The most commonly used model-based approach uses the Markov decision process (MDP), which is a general model of the environment in which the state is assumed to encapsulate all information necessary to predict the future (the *Markov* assumption). *Dynamic programming* is a classical search algorithm that can be used in an MDP to guide the agent towards a goal, which can be to optimise the agent's long-term reward [35]. *Q-learning* is the simplest model-free approach, and many variants of it have been proposed, mostly focussed on efficiency gains. The basic text on MDPs is Puterman(1994) [36]. Q-learning, as well as other model-free and model-based RL approaches are covered in Sutton and Barto (1998) [27].

Central to the problem of RL is the exploration/exploitation tradeoff. An RL agent can either exploit its current knowledge of reward (e.g., it may know of a particular action that will yield a good outcome) or it can try something new by exploring a new action that it has not yet tried. The first

2.3. OVERVIEW OF AI PRINCIPLES 21

option is safe while the second carries some risk, but may potentially yield a higher overall reward. Many RL agents use heuristic methods to trade-off exploration and exploitation. For example, an RL agent may try a random action some percentage of the time, slowly decreasing this percentage as it learns more and more about the environment. Another alternative is *optimism in the face of uncertainty* in which an agent always assumes an untested action is best. This approach is often very effective (fast) for RL but can carry more initial risk. Bayesian reinforcement learning (BRL) explicitly quantifies uncertainty over this tradeoff and is the optimal method for RL, but carries a significant computational overhead [37]. Efficient methods for BRL are a topic of much current research in the field of computer science.

2.3.3 MODELING INTERACTIONS BETWEEN USERS AND ZETs

When designing new ZETs it is important to first understand the types of interactions that may occur between the system and the user(s). In addition, the system needs to take into account various aspects of these interactions and other aspects of the context within which the system will be used. These aspects are critical as they will determine how best to model the variables that are related to the user, activity, and the environment and they will direct the appropriate choices of sensing and ML approaches. The following discussion presents an overview of some of the key variables that should be considered when developing sensing and ML algorithms for ZETs.

Uncertainty
The world is full of uncertainty, and healthcare and rehabilitation are no exception. Uncertainty becomes an even larger issue when deploying technologies into the homes and communities of potential users, which are typically highly unconstrained, dynamic, and unpredictable environments. Sources of uncertainty include noise from sensors, unobservability of events and states, and uncertain effects of actions. The latter is particularly important when working with people with disabilities, whose behaviours are sometimes difficult to predict, especially when supporting people with cognitive impairments. For example, when assisting a user during a self-care task, an assistive system needs to sense what the user is doing using some combination of sensors. These sensors carry with them explicit uncertainty, which will sometimes providing false readings. Further, the technology cannot directly measure various "hidden" states such as a user's awareness, level of frustration, or responsiveness to prompts. Finally, a user's abilities and reactions to the system may not always be predictable (i.e., they may change from day-to-day or over time), even though the user may be completing the same task within the same environment. A system that accounts for this uncertainty will be able to make better decisions than one that does not. A reading from an unreliable sensor, for example, may lead the system to deploy a more reliable (but more expensive) sensor rather than taking action based on the first reading. The system must have a model of this reliability (uncertainty) if it is to make this choice.

Modelling uncertainty, however, comes at the cost of an increased complexity of the model, since it must take into account more factors. ML can play a significant role in helping to better model these various factors, thereby enabling a system to learn about a particular user, detect changes in his or her abilities, and adapt appropriately both in short and long term contexts.

Model complexity and uncertainty are treated at length by MacKay (2003) [25]. A general tool for modelling uncertainty is the Bayesian network (BN), and the decision network (DN - also known as an influence diagram), and their dynamic counterparts (when time is involved), the Dynamic BN (DBN) and dynamic decision network (DDN). A Markov decision process (MDP) is a particular type of DDN. More complete treatments of BNs and DDNs can be found in Koller (2009) [34].

Time
A person with a disability often does not need help just once, but rather will need it repeatedly, through different tasks, and at different times of the day. As such, any assistance provided by a ZET needs to be an ongoing interaction, requiring the system to build and maintain an explicit model of time and a history of the user. AI-based approaches typically model time in one of two ways: event-based and clock-based. Event-based approaches use events as delineations of time. For example, a person entering the kitchen denotes the start of a kitchen event that lasts until the person leaves the kitchen. These events may have even finer resolution, such as the person touching a water faucet, indicating the start of that specific sub-step of a task, such as handwashing. Event-based modelling is very intuitive and powerful, as it allows for hierarchical modelling of nested events and corresponds to human perceptions of time, therefore may be easier for developers to define and model. Event based modelling can also be more sensitive to different user's abilities, as it is less focused on how long it takes someone to complete a task (event), but rather it focuses on whether or not the task has been initiated/completed. Clock-based approaches are a special class of event-based modelling in which the only events are (regular) time intervals taken from a clock. In other words, the system samples the environment (sensors) and performs logic operations at predefined time intervals; the end of time interval, when data collection and operations are performed, is considered to be an event. The advantage of a clock-based approach is it removes the need to specify what an event is, as it will perform data sampling and analysis after each time interval regardless of what is occurring in the environment. A drawback of the clock-based approach is that there may be far too many (if the time interval is set too short) or too few (if the time interval is too long) events for a particular task, resulting in oversampling and analysis or missed real-time events in the environment.

Adaptivity
One of the primary reasons for using AI in the design of ZETs is to create systems that are flexible and adaptable. Different people behave in different ways when presented with the same situation. Humans are also dynamic, and change over time; how a person reacts to a situation may change from one day to the next. This is especially true for people with disabilities, as many disabilities are progressive and cause significant changes in a person's abilities over time (both in the short and long term). Therefore, ZETs must have the ability to detect changes in a user's abilities and be able to adapt to these changes over time.

2.3. OVERVIEW OF AI PRINCIPLES   23

The primary way to approach adaptivity is through *learning* and/or *inference*. Both approaches assume the model being used has some unknown parameters that govern how the model works. For example, an assistance system may model the probability that a user needs help with a specific task. Once the system knows this probability, it can better tailor its assistive actions to the user: it has adapted. The *learning approach* attempts to find an estimate for the parameters given a set of training data. This estimate is usually the one that results in the best description or explanation of the data. This can take the form of either the most likely parameter setting given the data, the most likely parameter setting given the data and some prior information, or the most probable *distribution* over parameter settings given the data. In machine learning, the first case is known as maximum likelihood (ML), the second case as maximum a-posteriori (MAP), and the third case as *Bayesian learning*. In the MAP or Bayesian approach, one needs to define a prior over the parameter or parameter distributions, encapsulating knowledge about the types of distributions that may be encountered in the population in question. The additional descriptive power of the model in a MAP/Bayesian approach usually comes at the cost of more complex learning, and is more general. Detailed analysis of both of these methods can be found in MacKay (2003) [25], Koller (2009) [34], and Bishop (2006) [24].

A related approach is to assume a discrete set of parameter values, and to characterize membership of the set with a label index (class variable). *Inference* can then be used to infer the value of this class variable, and thereby which parameter settings (from the discrete set) are best at describing the data. In the previous example, a factor that affects the probability of a user needing assistance could be cognitive impairment level (e.g., mild, moderate, or severe), or impairment type (e.g., cortical vs. sub-cortical). Some fixed parameters would govern how a user's need for assistance during task completion depends on these variables. The model can then be used to infer the person's level or type of impairment and the system can use this to change its response characteristics so that they complement the user's needs and abilities.

Abstraction
ZETs are commonly used to sense real world events, which often resulting a large quantity of data that comes from a variety of different sensors. For example, a system assisting a person to complete a self-care activity might contain large volumes of raw data captured using video, switches, and other sensors to detect the user's hand and body positions and interactions with various objects. The data may also contain extraneous data that are irrelevant to the task at hand. Furthermore, video-based data are often collected with high frequency (typically around 10 to 30 frames per second) to ensure the system can detect changes in the user and environment. Even with a simpler type of sensor, such as a switch, the raw data emanating from it will be sampled at a rate that could provide a large amount of data over a period of hours, days, weeks, or years. As such, ZETs need to be able to sift through all of these data, and create appropriate abstractions of it, both in time and in space, and over a range of sensors. Moreover, in a continuous application (i.e., the instalment of a ZET in an environment for an indefinite period of time), it is important that the ZET is able to compact or

cull the data over time. Abstractions of classes or categories are critical in order to allow for simple and fast decision making for actions by the system.

In ML there are two primary techniques that are for creating and learning appropriate abstractions: generative and discriminative. *Generative techniques* attempt to model the complete distribution over all the sensor data by learning a function that maps between the abstract categories or classes and the raw sensor data. This function typically is very large and complex and can be quite difficult to learn. *Discriminative techniques* attempt only to find a method for classifying the data into the necessary categories, without worrying about the complete distribution of the data. A simple example is a water flow impeller in a pipe to detect if a person has turned on the water. A generative approach will build a function describing the distribution of sensor readings for each situation: water on or off. The distribution might take some parametric form, such as a Gaussian, or might be described by a nonparametric form, such as a histogram of values the sensor reading normally takes on for each of the states of the water flow. A discriminative approach will find the threshold for the sensor's output that will be the best predictor of the water being on or off. It should be noted that in theory, a generative modeling approach will always outperform a discriminative one if it is a correct model (if it is expressive enough) and if enough training data are available to learn the model. In practice, discriminative techniques offer better performance in terms of classification, particularly when only limited training data are available. Bishop (2006) [24] provides a comprehensive overview of both types of approach.

Specification and Preferences
An important aspect in developing ZETs is to ensure that the system aligns as closely as possible to the preferences and needs of the user. This aspect of *specification* involves two related problems: (i) specification of the machine-interpretable model of the interaction between the user, system, and task for which a person needs assistance, and (ii) specification of a user's *preferences* over the various outcomes. Typically, the first task is approached by engineers who gather information about the task and convert it into a usable model for assistance, while the second is approached by human factors specialists who gather information from end users about the relative worth of the various outcomes (as described later in this lecture in Section 3.1.2 on *User-Centred Design*).

The model specification involves the relationships between various elements of the task (including dynamics over time) and the user (their abilities, for example), and between the task and the sensors that are used to gather information from the environment. Engineers can usually gather this information and encode it in an appropriate model, but each new task requires substantial re-engineering and re-design to produce a working system. The automatic generation of such systems can substantially reduce the manual efforts necessary for creating and tailoring the systems to specific situations and environments. In general, the use of a-priori knowledge in the design of ZETs is a key unsolved research question. Researchers have looked at specifying and using ontologies [17], information from the Internet [38], logical knowledge bases [39], [40], and programming interfaces for context aware human-computer interaction [5].

2.3. OVERVIEW OF AI PRINCIPLES 25

The SNAP system [41] tackles this problem by starting with a description of a task and the environment that is relatively easy to generate. Interaction Unit (IU) analysis [42], a psychologically motivated method for transcoding interactions relevant for fulfilling a certain task, is used for obtaining a formalized, i.e., machine interpretable task description. This is then combined with a specification of the available sensors and effectors to build a working model that is capable of analyzing ongoing activities and assisting someone. The resulting model is called a SyNdetic Assistance Process or SNAP. A SNAP is a Partially Observable Markov Decision Process (POMDP—see Section 2.3), the specification of which is reduced to the IU task analysis complemented by the specification of a few key probabilities (e.g., the probability a person will respond to a prompt if given, or the probability the person will lose awareness in a task) and utilities (numerical encodings of a user's preferences – see below). Current work on SNAP is to provide an easy-to-use online interface for secondary end-users who are familiar with the tasks a person is needing assistance with, but unfamiliar with the complexities of the AI models used to build the automated assistance system This novel approach helps coping with a number of issues, such as validation, maintenance, structure, tool support, association with a workflow method, etc., which were identified to be critical for tools and methodologies which could support knowledge engineering for systems that plan and act in an environment.

The second aspect of specification is *preference elicitation* (PE). Key to any ZET is the encoding of the preferences of a user. These preferences may be as simple as a list of things that a person likes or does not like (e.g., he or she doesn't like audio prompts in a male voice), may be more complex (e.g., he or she likes audio prompts when in the kitchen, but not in the bathroom), or may be relational (e.g., likes audio prompts better than video prompts). Note that the specification of preferences is distinct from the model specification discussed above (e.g., using SNAP). Model specification simply defines the ways in which a user *can* or *normally will* interact with a system or environment, whereas preference specification encodes what the user really *wants* or *desires*. Preferences can therefore encode things outside the system (e.g., the user does not like any outcome suggested by the system, but perhaps has another, unknown outcome they are striving for).

While it is important for designers of ZETs to incorporate these preferences during the design phase, it is also critical for the technology itself to be able to extract this information during the operation of the system to ensure that the changing needs of the user are met. In machine learning, this can be achieved through the concept of *utility*, which can map a user's preferences onto a numerical utility function. Utility concepts originate in the study of game theory, operations research, and decision theory. Essentially, game theory guarantees that a rational human's preferences can be mapped onto a numeric scale of utility (i.e., the outcomes a person prefers will have a higher utility) and that decisions made according to this numeric scale will be the best, or optimal, for that person. However, it is known that humans do not always act rationally, and this may be even more apparent in a population of users with a cognitive disability. The study of preference elicitation (PE) – how to extract meaningful preference information from users – is an open research problem, but recent advances have allowed for its application in a variety of domains [43]. Recently, the fields of *imitation learning, apprenticeship learning, transfer learning,* and *inverse reinforcement learning* have come to the fore in artificial intelligence research as methods for approaching this problem, as described in more detail in the Spring 2011 issue of AI Magazine. These methods attempt to learn user preferences by observing a teacher, or by transferring learned preferences from other tasks.

In general, specification is closely tied to learning (as described previously), as the models and the preferences can change over time, and learning must be used to adapt these elements as the users and environments change. The specification task is one which is typically seen as taking place before any deployment, but can also be interleaved with actual use (e.g., a caregiver, as secondary user, may refine the model while it is not being used, or the user may explicitly change their preferences).

Experimental Performance

All the techniques presented thus far rely on some sort of training data. However, the actual aim of the learning process is to provide accurate classifications when the system is presented with data it has not seen before. That is, a classifier that does well on training data is not generally useful, as developers know the dataset (what the labels are, for example) and can manipulate the algorithms being used until the system is able to correctly classify this data. A recurrent problem in machine learning is that of overfitting, in which a classifier is trained on a static set of training data, on which it learns to perform very well (e.g., predict the labels), but then fails to perform well on test data. The model in such a case is too specific and usually overly complex in the sense that the classifier has modeled the training data too closely and, therefore, does not generalise well to real-world applications where the data may well be different. For example, if a vision-based system to recognise when a person is sitting in a chair is trained using only one type of chair, it will likely fail to recognise chairs that have a different design.

Avoiding overfitting is an art in itself that requires the model designer to carefully select the parameters to be learned so that they reflect the complexity and application of the classification problem appropriately. A simple technique for testing for overfitting involves separating the training data into two sets: a training set and a validation set. The machine learning algorithm is then applied to the training set then is evaluated on the validation set. The classifier that performs best on the validation set is the one that is most likely to generalise the best to other data. In practice, only a fraction (e.g., 10%) of the data set is needs to be reserved for validation. While testing a model using the validation method described above can be a good indicator of model generalisability, it is important to consider that the validation data may closely resemble the training data. For example, a data set for the chair recognition problem may contain images of many different types of chairs. However, if all the images were captured at the same angle, the classifier may do well on the validation data, but not perform well when implemented into a real-world environment. Therefore, developers must carefully select training data to ensure that it represents what the system would encounter in a real-world application as much as possible. A complete technical treatment of model selection and overfitting can be found in MacKay (2003) [25].

CHAPTER 3
Designing ZETs

With the above discussion about machine learning in mind, it is easy to see why it is crucial for ZET designers to gain a good understanding of the problem area and application parameters prior to developing any machine learning components. As is discussed in the next section, understanding and defining the problem scope may necessitate consulting with experts from other fields, such as clinicians, caregivers, and the intended end users of the system.

As noted in the previous sections, it is vital that every ZET is designed in a way that ensures it meets the needs and abilities of the people (or population) that will be using it. The principles of pervasive computing, artificial intelligence, and machine learning allow for sophisticated features and functions to be implemented into a ZET, however, this does not ensure that the resulting technology will be useful or accepted. In other words, while a device may be able to correctly interpret and react to environments and users, it also must be usable and effective from the perspective of the people using it. It is a lack of usability, and thus satisfaction, that often results in the abandonment or outright rejection of a technology by a user. To help mitigate this potential negative outcome, designers of ZETs need to be aware of practices and paradigms that can be used to gain an understanding of potential users and to build devices that complement their needs and abilities. Gaining a good understanding of potential users will also enable developers to collect targeted data that can then be used to build more effective and efficient AI algorithms.

3.1 COMMON DESIGN PARADIGMS

When designing for people with disabilities there are a variety of approaches that can be used to ensure that the resulting technology or system is usable by and appropriate for the targeted user(s). These approaches range from designing technologies to match the needs of a specific group(or type) of user who have similar abilities, to designing technologies that are intended for use by a broad group of people with varying abilities and needs. The two most commonly used paradigms—i.e. ideas underlying the methodology applied in a particular subject, in the development of ZETs are universal design and user-centred design. It is important to note that, as with most general principles and paradigms, universal design and user-centred design are concepts. As such, it is unlikely that any device can achieve full compliance because of unavoidable design conflicts. For example, situations may arise where two conflicting goals cannot be reconciled and a tradeoff must be made. Therefore, designers should use these concepts as a guide to gain a deeper understanding of the problem and application, identify potential conflicts in desirable outcomes, carefully weigh tradeoffs, and strive to achieve the best possible outcomes.

3.1.1 UNIVERSAL DESIGN

The goal of *universal design* (UD) is to create products and environments that can be used and experienced by people of all ages and abilities, to the greatest extent possible [44]. In the context of ZETs, developers try to apply the principles of UD to create a technology that can be used by as many different people as possible with as little adaptation or learning as possible. This concept does only apply only to developing a technology that can be used across different individuals, but also to developing the technology so that it can be used/operated by the user and his/her caregivers, family members, etc. Often the latter is a more important application of UD to ZETs and other assistive technologies. In the best examples, UD features go unnoticed because they have been fully integrated into design solutions that are used by a full spectrum of the population, including men, women, children, older adults, and people with disabilities. UD will also incorporate all of the accessibility features that are recommended or required by standards, codes, and legislation, however, in the most successful applications, these features are often not noticeable as they blend into the overall design [44]. The key concept of UD is that it is not an outcome of a design task, but rather it is a process and mindset that is used throughout the design process.

The term 'Universal Design' was first coined by Ronald Mace at North Carolina University, where he was the founding director of the Center for Universal Design. From its early definitions, UD was further developed by the Center to include seven principles as described below. The goals of these principles are to provide designers of products and environments with a set of objectives that can be easily followed and implemented into any design process, as well as a simple tool that can be used to validate a design with respect to whether or not it is accessible and usable by a wide range of individuals. While these principles were initially developed primarily for environmental design, such as architecture and landscape design, they are starting to be more applicable in the development of physical products and computer-based systems, such as ZETs, as well as non-tangible products, such as graphic design and communications [44].

Principle One: Equitable Use

The principle of *equitable use* states that a design should be useful and marketable to people with diverse abilities. Specifically, the design needs to provide the same means of use for all users; identical whenever possible, equivalent when not. Furthermore, the design must attempt to avoid segregating or stigmatizing any user as a result of an impairment, disability, or handicap, which necessarily includes making proper and equally effective provisions for safety and security. Finally, the first principle stipulates that a design should be appealing to all users with respect to aesthetics, materials, installation, etc.

Principle Two: Flexibility in Use

The second principle, *flexibility in use*, is aimed at ensuring that a design accommodates a wide range of individual preferences and abilities. This includes providing a choice of how a user can interact with a product or environment, such as accommodating left and right handed access and use, facilitating

3.1. COMMON DESIGN PARADIGMS   29

users' differences in accuracy and precision, and providing adaptability to different learning styles and paces. The latter is especially important when designing systems that are specifically for users with cognitive or learning disabilities.

Principle Three: Simple and Intuitive Use
The principle of *simple and intuitive use* states that a technology or system must be easy to understand and use, regardless of the user's experience, knowledge, language skills, or cognitive abilities. This notion is inline with an aforementioned goal of pervasive computing and ZETs, which is to reduce or eliminate the learning that is required to use a new technology. Simple and intuitive use is accomplished by reducing or eliminating unnecessary complexity, being consistent with user expectations and intuition, accommodating a wide range of literacy and language skills, and providing effective prompting and feedback during and after task completion.

Principle Four: Perceptible Information
The *perceptible information* principle builds upon the concept of providing effective prompting and feedback to a user by ensuring that the design communicates necessary information effectively to the user, regardless of ambient conditions or the user's sensory and cognitive abilities. Specifically, the design or system should use different feedback modalities (e.g., pictorial, verbal, tactile, etc.), maximize the probable uptake of essential and critical information, and provide compatibility with a variety of techniques or devices that a person may already be using, such as an assistive technology.

Principle Five: Tolerance for Error
The fifth principle, *tolerance for error*, states that a design needs to minimize hazards and potential adverse outcomes that may result from accidental or unintended actions. The design should arrange elements (e.g., buttons, controls, handles, and stairs) in a way that minimizes hazards and potential errors, provides clear warnings of potential hazards or errors, provides fail-safe features, and discourages unconscious actions that could be hazardous.

Principle Six: Low Physical Effort
The *low physical effort* principle states that the design must be able to be used efficiently and comfortably with a minimum amount of fatigue. This can be achieved by allowing a user to maintain neutral body postures, use reasonable operating forces, and require few or no repetitive actions. This principle can be extended to include low cognitive effort in order to accommodate those users with cognitive or intellectual disabilities. The principle of low physical effort is at the heart of many assistive technologies and ZETs, as these devices are specifically designed to make everyday tasks easier for people, both with and without disabilities.

Principle Seven: Size and Space for Approach

The seventh and final principle, *size and space for approach*, is focussed primarily on the environment within which a person may be completing a task, such as operating a technology or system. It states that appropriate size and space is provided for approach, reach, manipulation, and use regardless of the user's body size, posture, or mobility. This includes providing users with a clear line of sight to important elements and ensuring that adequate space is provided for the users who have assistive technologies (e.g., a wheelchair) or personal assistance (e.g., a caregiver).

3.1.2 USER CENTRED DESIGN

Often, ZETs and other technologies for health cannot be designed so that they are useable, and/or useful by the general public as they need to be able to perform highly specialized functions. Designers need to consider their primary user(s) and how their particular capabilities may impact their ability to effectively and safely use the technology being developed. This approach is known as *user-centred design* (UCD), which is a broad term to describe design processes where (representative) end-users and experts in different fields influence how a design takes shape [45]. UCD aims to create technology that identifies and meets the targeted users' needs as fully as possible, which can range from a single person to the general public, depending on the application. UCD is a general methodology and is commonly used in engineering design and human-computer interaction. It has been characterized by four activities, as described by Gould and Lewis [46] and later expanded upon by Wickens [47]:

1. seeking to understand user characteristics early in the design process;

2. adopting empirical techniques such as questionnaires, interviews, observations and focus groups to do so;

3. applying an iterative design-and-test cycle; and

4. employing participatory approaches in which users are, to varying degrees, involved in the design process.

Within UCD there is a wide variety of techniques and ways in which users are involved in the development of the technology, but the important elements of this paradigm are that users are involved one way or another and that the designers actively take into account the special needs and characteristics of the targeted users (for example to help with preference elicitation as previously described in the section on machine learning techniques).

UCD can be implemented based on a variety of approaches. For example, Norman (2002) proposed four primary recommendations to ensure that the user is always at the centre of the design [45].

- Make it easy for the user to determine what actions are possible at any moment.

- Make things visible, including the conceptual model of the system, the alternative actions, and the results of actions.

- Make it easy for the user to evaluate the current state of the system.

- Follow natural mappings between intentions and the required actions, between actions and the resulting effect, and between the information that is visible and the interpretation of the system state.

In a similar approach, Preece et al. (2002) describe the concept of *interaction design*, which is defined as "designing interactive products to support people in their everyday and working lives" [48]. Their process involved four basic activities:

1. identifying needs and establishing requirements;

2. developing alternative design that meet those requirements;

3. building an interactive version of the design so that it can be communicated and assessed;

4. evaluating what is being built throughout the process.

These activities are intended to inform one another and then be repeated as necessary [48].

Applying these various models and concepts, the role of the designer is to facilitate a task for the user and to make sure that the user is able to make use of the product as intended with a minimum level of effort to learn how to use it. This concept is applicable not only to the final product, but to all stages of the development and prototyping process as well.

The UCD process begins by discovering the users' requirements, which are used to compile the functional specifications of the device. This step often needs to be revised several times throughout the development process as the device's design evolves [49]. Discovering users' needs necessarily involves actual users and often has users performing tasks or activities in the environment(s) where they would use the technology. It is important for developers to remember that there are often several different users of a technology that go beyond the targeted main end-user. For example, a ZET that is designed to monitor and support a person with a chronic health condition may also be used directly or by proxy by his or her caregiver and clinicians. Each user type, and indeed each individual user, may have quite different opinions about what information and functionalities are beneficial, as well as how these data should be presented, who should be able to see the data, and how the user should interact with the system.

There are three different types of users that need to be considered in the UCD design process: primary, secondary, and tertiary [50]. Primary users are the people who actually use the device. Secondary users are those will occasionally use the device or those who use it through an intermediary, such as a caregiver having to help a person use their particular device. Tertiary users are people who will be affected by the use of the device or make decisions about its purchase, but do not use the device themselves. The inclusion of these different types of users is especially important in healthcare as the needs and expectations of a user's family members, caregivers, clinicians, and other health practitioners may also have to be taken into account. This is especially true in situations where the primary user is not making the decision to purchase a specific technology or is not the one paying for the device (as is often the case with technologies that support someone who has a disability).

Once the users and other stakeholders have been identified, information about their needs and preferences need to be collected in a systematic way through methods that may be structured, unstructured, or both [49]. Gathering structured information from users can take many different forms, such as questionnaires and interviews, formal measurements of users performing a specific task, and physiological measurements. Unstructured approaches may include comments made by users during an evaluation and observations made by developers. Structured data usually provides details about physical specifications, such as dimensions for components, while the unstructured data provides insight into preferences and can identify approaches that developers may not have considered.

A key component of the UCD approach is to develop several iterative prototypes of a technology and to evaluate it with the identified users and stakeholders as often as possible. The number of prototypes that will be needed depends on the project and technology being developed, however, UCD literature commonly recommends building and evaluating a minimum of three prototypes before deploying a technology into real-world applications [49]. The first prototype is used to present the concept of the device to potential users, to gather user feedback on initial ideas, and to generate potential alternative or additional functionalities and interface modalities. As it is intended for investigating a concept, first prototypes are usually put together quickly and without unnecessary complexity; these prototypes will typically be paper mock-ups and/or simple diagrams to demonstrate conceptual capabilities of the device, such as interfaces, data flow, and form factors. The second prototype incorporates what has been learned from the first evaluation to produce something that demonstrates more of the features of the proposed solution, but is not yet fully functional. Second level prototypes commonly employ a "wizard-of-oz" approach [51], where the developer simulates aspects of the technology (e.g., the reaction of the device to a person making an error during a task) using button presses or simple scripts to demonstrate possible functionalities of the device. Evaluations with the second prototype will result in further details about the problem and the effectiveness of the new solution. With the knowledge gained from second level prototype trials, the greater time and resources required to create prototypes that have a level of detail and functions that are akin to what would be seen in the final product. The third and subsequent stages of prototypes are appropriate for in-depth, long-term clinical trials that are conducted in real-world situations with actual users to ensure the efficacy of the system and to help build a case for technology transfer and commercialization.

3.1.3 INCORPORATING PRIVACY IN THE DESIGN PROCESS

As presented in the discussion of pervasive computing principles, ensuring that appropriate security and privacy features are built into the design of any ZET is extremely important as these technologies gather and transmit potentially sensitive data about users. The application of sensors and related technologies to the provision of healthcare and rehabilitation brings additional factors to the already complex issue of health information privacy [52]. Being able to ensure the privacy and security of user information will be a key determinant of the success of ZETs and other healthcare technologies.

In response to the trends toward the autonomous capture and transmission of data, the Information and Privacy Commissioner of Ontario, Canada developed a guideline in the mid-1990s that outlines the concept of *Privacy by Design (PbD)*. PbD entails embedding privacy into technologies beginning from the conceptualisation of the device, right through to commercialisation, retail, and ongoing operation and support [52]. In conjunction with PbD is the notion of a *positive-sum paradigm*, whereby privacy, a user's well-being, and commercialisation of a device may all be supported if privacy safeguards are proactively built into a system from the outset [52]. This paradigm has been well received in the pervasive computing and ZET fields, and indeed, many researchers have made the argument for the necessity of creating positive-sum PbDtechnologies. For example, Coughlin et al. (2007) found that the concerns of older adults with regard to smart home technologies included usability, reliability, privacy, and trust, among others. The study reported that pervasive systems would only be accepted if these issues were addressed right from the start [53]. Research by Kotz et al. (2009) described the goal of any remote health monitoring technology should be to develop usable devices that respect patient privacy, while also ensuring data quality and accessibility for the outcome of improved health [54]. Corporations such as Microsoft and Apple have acknowledged the importance of PbD and claim to support its use in their products.

Six principles have been developed to help designers of ZETs and other technologies ensure that the positive-sum PbDparadigm is met. Adhering to these principles helps designers to intrinsically incorporate privacy and security into a device throughout the design process, which is almost always more efficient and effective than attempting to address these issues in the final sages of development. The six principles are outlined below and more details about these principles and the PbD process can be found in [16].

Be proactive, not reactive

The first PbD principle is to *be proactive not reactive* in the implementation of privacy features in any new technology by anticipating and preventing as many privacy issues as possible before they happen. The identification and prediction of possible privacy concerns users might have can be achieved through the employment of the various techniques described in Section 3.1.2, such as user interviews, focus groups, and other human factors techniques (e.g., role playing, simulations, etc.). Designers must also be aware of best practices regarding the secure handling of data and incorporate protocols that ensure the data that are captured, analysed, and transmitted by the system are handled appropriately.

Privacy as the default

The second principle is *privacy as the default*, which seeks to deliver the maximum degree of privacy by ensuring that the default setting of the system is the one that ensures the maximum level of security. Put another way, a user should not be required to do anything in order to "turn on" privacy features in a system, rather the user should have to clearly and explicitly turn off any privacy features he or she feels are superfluous. Again, the technology designer needs to have a good understanding of the privacy and security features that should be in place by default, which settings can be deactivated by the user if they choose to do so, and what minimum level of security is required (regardless of any settings the user chooses) to ensure the data is handled in a way that is secure and compliant with relevant regulations.

Privacy is embedded into the design
The third principle is that *privacy is embedded into the design*. This means that privacy features must not be add-ons or are included after the initial system is designed; they must be integrated into the architecture of any ZET and the associated system support and business practices. The result of this principle is that privacy becomes an essential component of the core functionality delivered by the technology, without compromising operability.

End-to-end lifecycle protection
The fourth principle is *end-to-end lifecycle protection*. This principle advocates embedding privacy and security into the system prior to the first element of data being collected and to maintain privacy and security throughout the entire lifecycle of the data involved. This ensures that at the end of a system process (e.g., from data capture through the transfer of data from a home to a clinic, where after it is discarded), all data are handled and destroyed in a secure fashion.

Visibility and transparency
The fifth principle is *visibility and transparency*, which seeks to assure all stakeholders that a technology is operating according to the parameters stated by the technology's designers, researchers, and manufacturers. Furthermore, this principle includes a process for independent verification or audits to be made with respect to the security and privacy standards of the system. This principle is becoming an important aspect in the design and deployment of ZETs as these technologies are becoming more widespread and often handle sensitive data, therefore they are being subjected to increasing scrutiny from research ethics boards and governmental safety boards and associations (e.g., FDA, CSA) to ensure they employ appropriate security and privacy measures.

Respect for user privacy
The final PbD principle is *respect for user privacy*. This principle describes the essence and motivation for PbD as, above all, PbD requires system designers and operators to keep the interests of the individual at the forefront of the design process. Respect for users' privacy can be accomplished by implementing measures such as strong privacy defaults, the ability for a user to learn about what measures are in place should they wish to do so, clear and appropriate notice of any changes to security or privacy settings, and the implementation of user-friendly options.

3.1. COMMON DESIGN PARADIGMS 35

Applying PbD to ZETs

The concept of PbD can easily be applied in the design and development of new ZETs. As per the user-centred design approach, the central concept in PbD is to focus on the user and his or her needs and preferences with respect to security and privacy issues. Privacy-friendly defaults, appropriate notice, and user-friendly options and interfaces in ZETs are important to ensure that the user can fully engage in the protection and control of his or her own personal information. Systems' functionality should be transparent and their components visible, particularly in the application of ZETs to home health care scenarios. For example, individuals who are being monitored by a ZET should always be aware of where the sensors are installed, what data is being collected, and who can access it. Moreover, users should be able to participate in this process, playing an active role in choosing what devices are installed and explicitly stating who should have access to resulting data.

Privacy and security options should be available to users (and any designated representatives) at all phases of their relationship with the device and the device provider, which includes prior to installation, during the initial evaluation of the technology, and while the device is operating on a day-to-day basis [52]. Inline with the design approaches discussed in previous sections, engagement with users can and should begin at the initial design stages. Identifying potential privacy concerns at a conceptual stage of design allows PbD to be applied as a technology is being built, creating the possibility for discussions regarding user requirements during development. Moreover, incorporating privacy and security into each phase of the design process is generally easier and more effective than attempting to implement these practices post-hoc. Design practices used in the ZET field need to build complete visibility and transparency into systems by having representative users involved throughout the design process, by testing the final technologies, and by providing education sessions on how the system operates. This approach ensures that the system's users have an understanding of how a system operates and that reasonable and appropriate measures to protect privacy have in fact been incorporated into the final design [52]. Contrary to what one might expect, system transparency provides assurances that a person's privacy is being respected. Moreover, affording the user a measure of control over his or her own data fosters trust in the device, promotes active participation in device use, and decreases the likelihood of device abandonment.

Once the user's privacy requirements have been determined, the next stage of applying the PbD principles is in the design of the ZET system itself. This requires a number of privacy protections appropriate to the sensitivity and identifiably of the data and should be developed and proactively incorporated into the ZET. Given the (often) remote installation (e.g., a system running in a home rather than a clinical environment) and sometimes limited connectivity of the sensors themselves, it is important and far more effective in the long run to address all foreseeable privacy issues before they occur, as a breach in privacy would require updating or re-instrumenting a system after installation [52]. Wherever possible, protections should be embedded deeply into system components. For example, it may be possible to perform a great deal of data processing within the ZET itself or on a local (e.g., in-home) processor, which can drastically reduce the amount of data that is transmitted and allows the system to de-identify and encrypt data more effectively prior to transmission. Data that is transmitted from a ZET can contain information as simple as a reading and a sensor ID, for instance. By not transmitting any information about the user, the type of sensor, what is being measured, or any other kind of index that might connect the data to an individual, the odds of an unwanted third party intercepting and interpreting data decreases significantly. ZETs should also be designed to respect the principle of data minimization, collecting only information that is required for the specified purpose. Data should not be collected, for instance, based on an undefined potential future usage or because a developer or provider is interested in collecting data that are not related to the application in question. It is also crucial that systems are able to recognise if they are being compromised and alert the user and/or provider.

Finally, privacy features should require no or minimal effort of the part of the user; after settings are selected, the user should not have to actively enforce his or her privacy choices. As stated earlier in this section, ensuring adequate privacy and security is particularly important for ZET applications in the healthcare domain. Most ZETs are designed to operate without the user(s) being consciously aware of the systems, rather individuals are meant to be able to go about their normal lives, with devices taking readings inconspicuously and providing assistance only when required. Security and privacy measures for these types of systems are no exception, in that they should support the user continuously and discretely with little or no effort on the part of the user.

An interesting area of consideration is ZETs and other technologies that are designed to assist people in the case of an emergency. If a system is running or being used during an emergency, it is likely beneficial if the system can actively assist in procuring help. At this time, data privacy is likely not to be at the forefront of the individual's mind, although the data that could be used to assist the person could potentially be quite sensitive. For instance, a vision-based system could be able to automatically transmit images of the accident to emergency services so a professional can assess the situation and relay information to response crews, resulting in a faster, more targeted response. However, many people may see the automatic transmission of such information as a gross invasion of privacy. How these sorts of situations are treated, who gets to make ultimate decisions regarding potentially life-threatening situations, and if there are times when an individual's preferences should be overridden in the interests in protecting his or her well-being are some of the issues regarding privacy and security in ZETs and other smart technologies that are being intensely debated by the public, technology designers, and governments. Regardless, privacy via embedded and by-default protections must be something that the individual can *expect* to be present and should be made aware of any exceptions, such as any differences in operation and data transfer during an emergency situation [52].

3.2 KEY DESIGN CRITERIA FOR ZETS

One of the challenges developers face is selecting the specific hardware and software that will be used in a ZET to fulfill the technology's goals. This can be a difficult task, since there is a plethora of approaches a designer could use to build each different aspect of a ZET, as has been alluded to in the previous sections. Matching components to the specific application and user(s) needs requires careful planning. This section presents eight ZET design criteria that have been developed by the authors based on the design paradigms presented earlier in this lecture and from the expertise of researchers in the field of smart technology development. These criteria are intended to "guide" technology designers who are working with special populations to ensure that the needs, preferences, and context of the user is taken into account. These principles are intended to be easily incorporated into any new ZET and are applicable to all the different aspects of a ZET, such as artificial intelligence, pervasive computing, privacy by design, and, above all, sensitivity to user needs.

3.2.1 DEVELOP FOR REAL-WORLD CONTEXTS

When designing ZETs, developers need to ensure that they are addressing a real-world need that is driven by the end user(s). Effective ZETs are not technology-driven. Instead, they seek to understand and implement the most appropriate technologies for supporting the needs of the user(s).

Many assistive technologies and other devices developed for healthcare and rehabilitation are not used. It is estimated that anywhere from 50–70% of all devices are abandoned post-implementation [55, 56]. One of the most highly cited reasons for abandonment is that the technology did not meet the actual needs of the user; the device did not enable the user to do the things they expected the device would help them do and/or the device was more trouble than it was worth. To avoid such pitfalls, ZET designers need to first understand the problem(s) for which they are developing a new technology to solve. This can only be achieved by a through understanding of the problem, the expectations of the end user(s), and the environment where the technology will be deployed. This understanding can be achieved through the use of the various techniques presented earlier in the lecture.

The first step in grounding the design process in real-world problems is to gain an understanding of the *context* for which the ZET is being designed. The *International Classification of Functioning, Disability, and Health* framework published by the World Health Organization [1] defines contextual factors as external environmental factors (e.g., social attitudes, architectural characteristics, legal and social structures, climate, etc.), and internal personal factors (e.g., gender, age, disease type, coping styles, and education). As all of these factors influence how the end user experiences disability, it is important that the designer gains insight into these various factors well before developing a new technology. Designers also need to be aware that the contextual factors that are important to one type of user may be different from those that affect a different user. As such, it is also important to identify which factors are of particular importance before entering into the design process. Once these contextual factors have been identified and understood, the designer can then begin to develop the algorithms and sensors needed to collect data and build the models necessary for the system to be able to operate effectively.

3.2.2 COMPLEMENT EXISTING ABILITIES

When creating ZETs, developers should focus on what the person is able to do and leverage these abilities to enable them to achieve what they cannot do.

The goal of ZETs, and indeed all technologies, is to enable people to do things they could not have done otherwise. While providing support in a manner that supplants a person's abilities may achieve the same result as one that complements abilities, the emotional and physical outcomes may be drastically different. Research has shown that engagement in one's surroundings can have a significant impact on slowing the decline in abilities [57]. Technologies that support and complement existing abilities enable a person to remain as interactive in his or her environment as possible, fostering control and independence. For instance, many older adults with dementia have difficulties with mobility but are not permitted to use powered wheelchairs as impairments in judgement and reaction time can make them dangerous drivers. In response to this need, researchers are taking different approaches to assisted mobility that range from anti-collision systems to fully autonomous navigation. While the latter may be suitable for people who have lost all mobility, it is erroneous to assume that older adults with dementia do not have the capacity to know where they want to go or how to operate their chair to get there. With a fully- or mostly-automated approach, the chair's occupant becomes little more than a passenger, placidly being conveyed to destinations with little control as to where they are going or how they get there, decreasing cognitive stimulation and control, which increases feelings of helplessness and apathy. On the other hand, intelligent chairs can be built that complement the driver's abilities to promote dignity and independence, such as a chair that can provide prompts to help drivers make decisions and the use of anti-collision devices to enable a person to go where they wish without the risk of hitting people or objects.

3.2.3 USE APPROPRIATE AND INTUITIVE INTERFACES

Interfaces that are simple, intuitive, and appropriate make technologies more accessible and useful to people with disabilities and their caregivers. Whenever possible these interfaces should be invisible to the user and naturally part of the user's existing environment and context.

Technologies designed for users with special requirements need to take into account a variety of impairments and comorbidities that include decreases in physical, cognitive, and sensory abilities. If a user interface is required, large displays, loud and clear audio cues, and simple, high contrast interfaces are some examples of appropriate designs for this population. While they may provide a convenient and adaptable interface, devices such as touch-screen cell phones may not be appropriate as they may be unfamiliar to some users, can be easily misplaced, and are potentially difficult or finicky to use. Technologies that are embedded into the environment that do not have explicit interfaces are often more appropriate as they do not require the user to remember to wear a device or change the way they go about their everyday lives. Moreover, embedded technologies maximise connectivity while minimising maintenance, such as changing batteries or accidentally damaging the device. Reacting to trends in the growing role of ambient monitoring in healthcare, most assisted living communities are being built to support embedded sensor technology with extra power, communication conduits, and removable paneling installed during construction, a trend that is starting to spread to the community in general.

3.2.4 ENCOURAGE INVOLVEMENT WITH THE USERS' ENVIRONMENT

Devices that encourage people with disabilities to interact with their environments help to stimulate interest in their surroundings and help them to relate with others.

Difficulties with motor skills, sensory losses, and decreases in executive memory tasks means that people with disabilities often experience a profound loss in control over their environments. Uncertainty and confusion frequently results in diminished or impaired physical and social involvement. Many ZETs are targeted toward ameliorating these losses through interventions that range from supporting activities of daily living to promoting social inclusion. For example, the CIRCA project has been designed to aid reminiscences in order to help people with dementia converse with family and caregivers [58]. The device consists of a touch screen that enables access to photos, music, video, text, and other materials that were selected by caregivers and psychologists to help people access memories. The tool has a friendly, simple interface that encourages people with dementia to interact with it and enables them to choose themes and media. As the interface is usable by the people with dementia themselves, they are able to decide which topics are selected and therefore are more likely to initiate and have control over the resulting conversations. Jimison et al. have developed algorithms that provide a dynamic, real-time assessment of seniors' cognitive abilities through tracking a user's performance on computer games, such as FreeCell and custom-built spelling and shape matching games [59]. These algorithms not only estimate the user's cognitive performance and identify changes over time, but can also use the data to autonomously adjust the difficulty level of the game to match the user's level of skill. These are examples of ZETs that encourage users to interact with the technology and their environment by complementing the users' abilities to provide usable and useful interfaces.

3.2.5 SUPPORT THE CAREGIVER

Support the caregiver to enable them to focus on tasks other than caregiving, thus reducing caregiver burden and enabling a better relationship with the care recipient.

Caring for someone with a disability is a very demanding task that results in a great deal of caregiver burden, which has been shown to cause high levels of stress, depression, and even an increased risk of mortality [60, 61]. A device that adds to caregiver burden is unlikely to be accepted as the caregiver is often already at the limits of his or her capabilities. Moreover, caregivers may have morbidities of their own to manage, which can make learning or using a complex technology an impractical alternative. Interventions should be robust and as autonomous as possible, requiring only simple and infrequent input from a caregiver. Ensuring the caregiver understands how a technology works, is supported by the technology, and does not need to invest effort in a technology will foster confidence and acceptance of the intervention. As such all of the design principles and criteria related to ZETs need to also be applied to the caregiver.

3.2.6 COMPLEMENT EACH INDIVIDUAL'S CAPABILITIES AND NEEDS

Artificial intelligence, machine learning, and decision making techniques have the potential to create technologies that are able to tailor themselves to the user's specific and individual abilities, enabling guidance that is appropriate, relevant, and effective.

Like any other person, users of ZETs have their own wishes and preferences about the type of technology they would like to use, how they would like to interact with a technology, and the form factor of the technology (i.e., what the technology looks like). Identifying these preferences is important, particularly for technologies that interact with the user (as opposed to passive monitoring). As people with various disabilities, especially cognitive impairments, are often unable to answer specific questions or perform specific actions, capturing and understanding preferences can be challenging as they are mostly inferred from observations over a period of time. In this respect, work in the field of preference elicitation is very valuable (see Section 2.3.3). The autonomous identification of preferences though observations of a person's actions complements the need for device personalisation and minimal explicit demands from the caregiver and care recipient. It is only through the identification and accommodation of user's individual needs that a technology becomes truly useful.

3.2.7 PROTECT THE USERS' PRIVACY AND ENABLE CONTROL OVER PREFERENCES

Devices should operate in a way that matches the user's information sharing preferences, needs, and abilities. The user (or his or her caregiver) should be able to easily change these settings at any time to match changes in circumstances.

Technology should be transparent so that it allows stakeholders (e.g., the primary user, his or her caregiver, family members, health practitioner, etc.) the ability to understand and have control over the data that are being collected, stored, and transmitted. A high-level understanding of what is going on inside the "black box" makes people feel more comfortable with the technology and therefore more likely to accept it. Moreover, implicit clarity and transparency about what the device is doing enables people to intuitively gauge the value of the assistance that is being provided to them and affords them the ability to adjust it to fit their needs, making it more applicable over the long-term. There is also a wide variability in peoples' comfort level toward what data is communicated. As such, users should have control over settings so that they can select the configuration of their choice.

3.2.8 ENSURE EXPANDABILITY AND COMPATIBILITY

It is important to ensure that ZETs are compatible with other types of technologies that a person currently uses and that, whenever possible, a ZET can be easily expanded to include other required functions.

Through the application of pervasive computing principles, ZETs should be able to operate as stand-alone devices or in tandem with other technologies and assistive devices. This capability allows consumers to pick which ZETs are appropriate for their particular needs and addresses the practical challenges associated with developing a single technology that can support multiple daily activities. The ability to combine data from multiple technologies also allows the creation of a richer and more holistic representation of the people they are supporting. This information can be used to provide targeted and tailored interventions to match the individual's needs and particular situations.

CHAPTER 4
Building and Evaluating ZETs

Guided by the methods described in the previous sections, such as *Wizard-of-Oz techniques*, device development is usually iterative in nature, becoming more involved as a product evolves. As discussed, development can be done in a modular fashion, with a number of sub-systems interacting to form the overall device. Each sub-system is usually responsible for a specific aspect of the device, such as sensor input or decision making, and communicates relevant data to the other sub-systems over a shared bus or network. This approach is flexible and allows designers to develop, integrate, and optimise sub-systems sequentially or in parallel without having to retool the entire device. It also allows sub-systems to be altered, adapted, upgraded to fit specific applications or to incorporate new algorithms or hardware that become available post-implementation.

Regardless of the approaches used to create or improve a ZET, developers should have measurable outcomes; a set of specific goals or objectives that the developer wishes to achieve. As they represent goals the design team wishes to achieve, measurable outcomes can be used to guide the direction of a technology's development, gauge performance improvements, and signal when milestones have been reached. Outcomes can be short-term or long-term, can be ranked in terms of importance, and may change over the course of the development process as a project's scope becomes more defined.

Importantly, outcomes should include non-technical measures of success, such as the device's impact on user independence and user satisfaction with the device. While these outcomes are often difficult to measure reliably and quantitatively, they are crucial (and the ultimate) measures of a device's success. For instance, even if a device operates flawlessly from a technical perspective, if users do not feel it is useful, or worse, if it causes users to become annoyed or frustrated, then it is not a successful intervention as it likely hinders rather than helps the user and will be rejected by the people it is intended to assist.

Depending on the resources, stage of development, and nature of the application, device developers may use some or all of the following techniques sequentially, in parallel, or iteratively throughout the design process.

4.1 IN SILICO TESTING

In silico testing consists of creating, debugging, and optimising a new technology in a virtual environment on a computer. The purpose of *in silico* testing is to create an operational model of the system as well as to identify and address as many issues as possible in a virtual environment before porting the system to a version that interacts with hardware. As the system is in a virtual environment, it has the advantage of being extremely malleable and allows developers to modify the system as they wish without having the added complications of having to ensure changes do not interface with hardware or interfaces. Another advantage to *in silico* testing is that there are no physical constraints to the system. Using this technique, different approaches can be investigated relatively easily and at a low cost prior to building a prototype. Indeed, the final virtual model that is selected may dictate hardware and interface choices. For instance, while a developer may have a particular application and associated hardware in mind, such as the type of sensor to be used, the development and testing of a system *in silico* can help to solidify specific physical deployment parameters.

As *in silico* testing uses explicit and known inputs, it is a powerful and effective method for adding new functionalities, targeting areas for development, debugging and optimisation, and investigating specific scenarios. Developers can run an identical input as many times as they wish, enabling the direct comparison of different versions or approaches to solving the same problem. For example, in computer vision applications, developers commonly use machine learning with large datasets of pre-recorded videos or images to train a system. Using the same dataset allows developers to try different machine learning techniques and to tune the application's parameters to optimise factors such as accuracy and computational efficiency, and balance tradeoffs, such as model complexity and precision versus generalizability and resources required. As previously described in the section on Artificial Intelligence, cross validation is a technique that is often employed, where a portion of a dataset is set aside to validate the model after it has been trained. With cross validation, the model is trained using the majority of the data set then tested using the reserved data to see if the system interprets input appropriately and accurately, enabling a developer to gauge the model's performance and applicability to the application.

Once a system model has been selected, developers often use button presses (e.g., using a keyboard or buttons), scripted code, or a sub-set of a dataset (as discussed above) to simulate input the device could experience if it were operating in the real world. Sometimes experts in a related field, such as clinicians, will be consulted to construct realistic test scenarios. This final step of *in silico* development can be used to further optimise a system before it is ported to a prototype.

4.2 BENCHTOP TRIALS

In benchtop trials, hardware and software are combined to form a functional version of a device that developers can interact with. The ability to interact with a device and its components adds a layer of complexity as the device's hardware and software are physically present, integrated, and, ideally, running in real-time. Benchtop trials allow developers to physically simulate scenarios in a manner that is representative of what the device would experience in a real-world application. Interacting with the device assists with the identification and tuning of numerous design requirements, such as the hardware selection, logistics concerning device assembly and installation, and the establishment of communication protocols between device components, sub-systems, and external services. Devices can be assembled piecemeal, with one portion or sub-system of a device assembled at a time. Often, the portions of a system that are not yet built can be simulated *in silico* and interact with the parts that are physically present.

Benchtop trials can range from testing the system and its components at a workstation, to testing in mock-ups of real environments. Many organisations have begun to use test smart homes to trial new devices in a simulated home environment, which can be used to test operability of a device on its own and can also be used to investigate how it integrates with other systems (both smart and otherwise). Through benchtop trials, a device transitions from the conceptualisation phase into an operational device.

4.3 ACTOR SIMULATIONS

While experienced developers may have a good understanding of the general behaviours and attitudes of the population they are designing for, these traits can be quite difficult to replicate authentically. Actors, however, have trained extensively to take specified emotions and attitudes to play specific roles. Role-playing by actors is often used to simulate conditions or situations of interest for teaching and assessments in medicine. This allows medical students to learn about specific scenarios and investigate the effects of treatment options prior to encountering them in a real patient. Similarly, actors have started to be used to optimise devices and assistive technologies. The use of actors allows developers to gain a better understanding of how a device is likely to be used and how it will react to the population of interest prior to deployment.

Using actors is a valuable and cost-effective option compared to testing solely through clinical trials (which are discussed below). Once actors are trained on examples of the population of interest, they can simulate scenarios consistently for as long as is needed. This is especially advantageous when the targeted user group is a vulnerable or frail population, such as older adults with dementia. Using actors allows data to be collected much more quickly, has a low ethical risk (as actors are cognitively aware, consenting adults), generally requires significantly less resources to complete, and allows for the emulation of specific scenarios. The ability for actors to replicate specific behaviours and scenarios gives developers the significant benefit of being able to test a device or system with more conditions than would likely be encountered using a small clinical trial or pilot study.

One study has tested the applicability of the use of actors to develop ZETs for older adults with dementia by having professional, older adult actors train on videos of people with dementia washing their hands [62]. The actors then emulated handwashing first guided by a human caregiver, then guided by COACH; a ZET that assists people with dementia through handwashing (as described in the next section). Professional caregivers were asked to watch videos of the actors shown and (previously captured) videos of older adults with dementia then asked to rate how believably the person in the video portrayed dementia. The professional caregivers gave similar believability ratings for both conditions. The actors also elicited reactions from COACH that were comparable to real older adults with dementia [62].

While using actors is a powerful method of prototype device debugging and optimisation, it must be made clear that this method is not intended to replace the need to test the device with real people from the target population(s). Rather, optimization using actors can dramatically improve device performance compared to benchtop trials alone, resulting in better performance in clinical trials and in the ultimate deployed system or device.

4.4 TRIALS WITH CLINICAL POPULATIONS

Trials with a representative group of users from the population(s) of interest are implemented in the later stages of the development process as they involve the device being tested with people and in the environments that they are designed to operate with. No matter how thoroughly a device is scrutinised prior to clinical trials, the technology will be confronted with a multitude of scenarios that have not yet been encountered. As such, it is only through the exposure to a representative sample of end-users and environments that developers can truly gauge how the technology will perform in the real world.

Clinical trials range from pilot studies in controlled environments to large-scale, long-term installations in peoples' homes. Conducting clinical trials is the most direct and comprehensive method of testing a device's capabilities and robustness, however, they are also usually far less supervised than other forms of device testing, therefore the device must be robust and functional prior to deployment.

While clinical trials are a crucial step in the development process, they are also the most complex and costly. A technology that is going to be used in a clinical trial should be optimised as much as is reasonably possible prior to the trials to maximise the likelihood of the technology's success. Trial methodologies should be carefully planned to ensure that trails run smoothly, that there are sufficient resources available to complete the trials, and that data is captured that allows for a critical and meaningful evaluation of the device's performance. It is important that clinical trials are well supported to ensure logistics are handled in a timely and professional manner, including equipment installation and removal, user education, and support in the case of device failure. Moreover, contingency support must be in place to ensure that no harm comes to trial participants should the technology fail, particularity if the device is intended to support a person's well-being. These demands can often result in a research team that is larger and from a greater diversity of backgrounds than the device development team. In particular, trials involving people with disabilities generally require special considerations and extra resources.

By and large, the challenges presented by clinical trials are outweighed by the opportunity for developers to gain a good understanding of how the device operates when it is deployed into the real world. The results and feedback gained through clinical trials can be especially helpful in identifying deficiencies, are very helpful in targeting future development efforts, and can provide the proof of efficacy required to transfer a device from the research and development phase to commercialisation.

CHAPTER 5

Examples of ZETs

Over the past several years there have been numerous technologies and systems developed for people with a wide variety of disabilities. As such, this section will only include examples of technologies that meet the previously stated definition of a ZET, specifically *technologies that employ techniques such as artificial intelligence and unobtrusive sensors to autonomously collect, analyse, and apply data about the user and their context.* In addition, the majority of these systems have been developed for people with cognitive impairments, as this population most likely will benefit the most from these types of technologies and the adaptability, guidance, and compensatory abilities that they may provide. As such, this section reflects the current trends in ZET development and focuses on devices to support people with cognitive impairments. The reader is referred to [63–66] for more information on intelligent technologies and systems that fall outside the scope of this lecture.

5.1 AREAS OF APPLICATION

The complexity and variability of a disability means that support must be appropriately sensitive, personalised, dynamic, robust, and context-aware. This can be especially true for people with a cognitive impairment, as users can lack the understanding or judgement required to identify and rectify a situation if the ZET provides sub-optimal guidance or, worse, makes a mistake. While the following have been identified as areas where ZETs can provide support for people with cognitive impairments and their caregivers, many of these areas translate to other populations, including the general public.

Safety: A cognitive impairment can often compromise a person's safety as they may not be able to anticipate or react to adverse situations appropriately. Monitoring a person can enable the detection of adverse events, such as the person falling or becoming ill, and procure assistance when required.

Long-term trend prediction: Monitoring a person over an extended period of time can be used to detect long-term trends in behaviour. Deviations in trends can indicate potential health problems or changes in cognition.

Assistance with daily activities: Being able to perform activities of daily living, such as bathing, toileting, and dressing, are crucial to maintaining independence. Difficulties with executive memory functioning often results in an inability to remember what steps are required to complete an activity or how to complete them. Supporting daily care activities can help to mitigate dependency on a caregiver.

Communication: Cognitive impairment can make interpersonal interactions difficult, causing feelings of isolation and depression. Technologies that assist in recollection and promote communication can enable meaningful interactions with people who have a disability.

Leisure: Participating in leisure for people to relax while simultaneously encouraging personal expression. Participation in activities such as artistic expression can provide a meaningful occupation for people with a cognitive impairment, increase their engagement with their environments, and provide an emotional outlet.

Cognitive stimulation: There is growing evidence that cognitive stimulation can help to slow the progression of impairment. Technologies that foster engagement could play a significant role in slowing cognitive decline and in the monitoring of cognitive abilities.

It should be noted that these areas are not mutually exclusive. As will be shown in the following examples of different technologies, one type of ZET can span more than one of these application areas.

5.2 OVERVIEW AND COMPARISON OF EXAMPLES

Table 5.1 summarises the systems described in this section, which represent various AI methodologies, pervasive computing devices, and areas of application. Regardless of the technical approach, all of the systems are intended to support users in their goals to interact with their environments; none are meant to provide fully automated, context-free solutions. As illustrated by Table 1 and follow-up detailed discussions of each technology, the majority of research in this field has focused on systems that help with ADL completion. In addition, many of these systems have been developed for adults or older adults with cognitive impairments, such as mild cognitive impairment or dementia. In terms of testing, several systems described in this section have undergone technical efficacy trials, however, once user tests are implemented, issues around intuitive interfaces, which is also a ZET design criterion, commonly arise. Some of these issues may be circumvented by adopting a user-centered approach that investigates user needs, preferences and environmental constraints upfront; others may only arise within real-life contexts and may prove impossible to foresee in simulation and lab testing. With respect to the other design criteria, significant variation exists between projects, particularly in areas of privacy and caregiver support, which have been consciously addressed in some projects, but unreported in others. Non-reporting suggests that these are principles that have yet to be universally implemented. However, in light of the recent emergence of this field, it is expected that as development of ZETs mature, these principles will increasingly be invoked.

5.3 AUTOMINDER

Autominder is one of the first ZETs that was developed to provide flexible and context-sensitive reminders to people who have trouble with memory tasks through the application of many of the AI techniques and sensors described in Chapter 2 [67, 68]. Autominder uses probabilistic approaches

Table 5.1: Overview and comparison of example ZETs developed for health, wellness, and rehabilitation. *Continues.*

Features	Autominder	COACH	Archipel	Assisted Cognition	PEAT
Application area	ADL support - Reminder system	ADL support - Hand washing	ADL support - Meal preparation	Safety - Directional guidance	ADL support - Reminder system
Target population	Adults with memory problems	Adults: cognitive impairment, dementia Children: autism	Adults with cognitive impairment	Adults with mild cognitive impairment	Adults with executive function impairment
Design paradigm	Simulation-based design	UCD approach	UCD approach	Scenario-based design	Scenario-based design
Input devices	Environmental sensors	Web camera	Environmental sensors RFID tags Touch screen	Wearable GPS unit GIS street map information	Wearable RFID bracelet Environmental sensors GPS sensor
Output devices	Robot (non-adaptive system) Handheld device (adaptive system)	Flat screen monitor Speakers	Flat screen monitor Lighting devices Speakers	GPRS-enabled cell phone	Cell phone
Machine learning - Reasoning	Reinforcement -Temporal constraint reasoning	Supervised -Probabilistic neural network and computer vision	Supervised / Reinforcement -Hierarchical Markov Model -POMDP	Unsupervised -Hierarchical Markov Model Dynamic Bayesian network	Unsupervised -Interleaved Hidden Markov Model, Propel AI

Table 5.2: *Continued.* Overview and comparison of example ZETs developed for health, wellness, and rehabilitation. *Continues.*

Features	Autominder	COACH	Archipel	Assisted Cognition	PEAT
Test Results -Test -Population -Description -Results	Preliminary field trials with *non-adaptive* unit. - older adults and adults with traumatic brain injury -prototype learned specific patterns 82% of the time. Simulation-based feasibility studies with adaptive unit. -simulated users and environment. - results: positive	Usability study -adults with moderate to severe dementia (n=10) -baseline vs prototype -prototype increased number of steps correctly performed without carer assistance by 25%	Usability study -adults with cognitive impairment (n=12) -baseline vs prototype -prototype reduced number of in-person cues	Indoor usability study -adults with cognitive impairments (n=6) -baseline vs prototype -positive results with usability issues Outdoor usability study -adults with cognitive impairments (n=9) -cues correctly followed 150 of 180 times	Simulation studies -simulated users -baseline vs prototype -appropriate cueing compared to baseline

Table 5.3: *Continued.* Overview and comparison of example ZETs developed for health, wellness, and rehabilitation. *Continues.*

Features	PROACT	ePAD	HELPER	Rehab Robotics
Application area	*Trend prediction* - Activity recognition	*Leisure* - Creative expression	*Safety* - Fall detection	*ADL support* - Rehab exercise
Target population	Adults with cognitive impairments	Older adults, people with demetia	Older adults	Adults, post-stroke
Design paradigm	UCD approach	UCD approach combined with participatory design	UCD approach	UCD approach
Input devices	Multi touch screen RFID-tagged objects RFID-tagged glove or bracelet Web camera	Multi touch screen Web camera	Web camera Microphone	Body sensors Virtual environment
Output devices	Activity prediction report	Flat screen Speakers	Speakers External phone line	Robotic device Haptic exercise **platform** Flat screen
Machine learning - Reasoning	Unsupervised -dynamic Bayesian network with Monte Carlo - based inference	Reinforcement -POMDP	Supervised -Support vector machines, neural networks, and computer vision	Reinforcement -POMDP with fuzzy logic intelligence

Table 5.4: *Continued.* Overview and comparison of example ZETs developed for health, wellness, and rehabilitation.

Features	PROACT	ePAD	HELPER	Rehab Robotics
Test results -Test -Population -Description -Results	Model validation study -healthy adults (n=14) -site: home fitted with RFID tags -precision: 88% overall (100% for 8/14 ADLs) -sensitivity: 73%	Usability study -older adults (n=6) -art therapists (n=6) -outcome measures: effectiveness, efficiency, satisfaction. -results forthcoming	Model validation study -healthy adults -7-day in-home trial -true positives: 100% -false positives: minimal	Pilot trials -therapist -users (n=8) -baselinevs prototype -device agreement with therapist: 65% -user satisfaction: positive

and supervised machine learning algorithms to model both what the person is doing and what the person should be doing. Autominder is not intended to give detailed instructions on how to complete a task, rather it is meant as a high-level reminder system. When a new task is scheduled with Autominder, the person inputting the task not only specifies when the task should happen, but can also specify a temporal tolerance for the task (i.e., an acceptable "window" for the task to be initiated, such as +/- 30 minutes from the scheduled time). Using this information, Autominder can give context-sensitive reminders to a person only if a person needs them (i.e., has not already completed the scheduled task). The overall architecture for the system is shown in Figure 5.1.

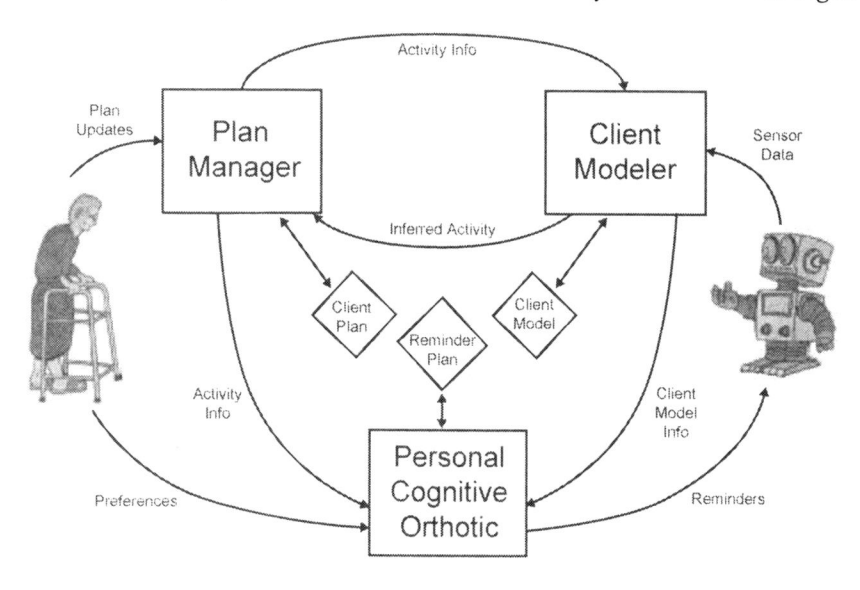

Figure 5.1: Autominder architecture showing the plan manager, client modeler and their interactions with the personal cognitive orthotic device.

The *Client Modeler* (Figure 5.1) employs environmental sensors and machine learning to learn about the user and his or her context (i.e., the user's preferences, what the user is doing, and the state of his or her environment) and combines this with the temporal tolerance of the task to deliver prompts at times when he or she may be the most effective. Determining the appropriate prompts and time of delivery is determined by the *Plan Manager* (Figure 5.1). For example, if a person is scheduled to take medication every day at 1 PM, but Autominder knows his or her favourite TV show is on at 1 PM on Wednesdays, on Wednesday Autominder may prompt the person to take his or her medication at 12:55 rather than delivering the prompt during the show, when it may be ignored or forgotten. Unlike a conventional reminder system, Autominder's context awareness means it will not provide a prompt to the user for a task he or she has already completed. This is important in supporting independence and minimising confusing messages (e.g., if a non-context aware system reminds a person to take medication they have just taken, it could result in a double-dose). These prompts are then delivered via some user interface, represented by the *Personal Cognitive Orthotic* (Figure 5.1), which can take a variety of forms, such as a mobile robot, or a handheld device.

Preliminary tests with older adults and people who have traumatic brain injury have shown promising results, although an in-depth evaluation has yet to be completed. Autominder was "…developed with four sometimes competing goals in mind: 1) user awareness of planned activities; 2) a high level of user and caregiver satisfaction; 3) avoiding introduction of inefficiency into the user's activities; and 4) avoiding over-reliance on the reminder system – that is, reliance to the extent that use of the system actually decreases rather than increase [the] user's independence" [68, p. 69]. These goals are an excellent and succinct example of design criteria for a ZET technology for people with cognitive impairments.

5.4 THE COACH

The COACH (Cognitive Orthosis for Assistive aCtivities in the Home) is an example of ZET designed specifically to help older adults with cognitive impairments (e.g., Alzheimer's disease) through common activities of daily living (ADLs). COACH's developers chose to initially focus on one ADL, handwashing, to enable them to gain a good understanding of the context and to investigate and implement appropriate ways of modelling the problem and providing appropriate support to users [69, 70]. As shown in Figure 5.2, the current version of COACH consists of a video camera mounted over the sink, a computer, speakers, and a flat-screen monitor. The overall architecture of the system is illustrated in Figure 5.3. Using computer vision, COACH tracks the user's hands, the towel, and the soap as he or she interacts with the sink area. This is achieved by using image processing techniques that learn the different characteristics of the user's hand (e.g., skin colour), and the other relevant objects (e.g., location). This information is passed to a planning module, which employs machine learning and inference techniques to determine autonomously where in the task the user is and to estimate parameters such as the user's overall level of dementia, current responsiveness, and preferred ordering of steps. The planning module then uses this information to decide the best course of action to take; namely, to continue to observe the user, give the user an audio or video prompt to guide him or her to the next step in the activity, or to summon the caregiver should the user require assistance.

COACH is a good example of a ZET as it does not require any explicit input from the user with dementia or the caregiver to make decisions and provide support autonomously. Importantly, the system follows the user through the task without the user having to wear any markers or other devices, avoiding possible non-compliance or annoyance from the person with dementia and also freeing the caregiver from needing to ensure the care recipient is wearing the tag or device, that it is charged, and that it is operational. COACH is able to learn about the user's preferences and is able to change its short- and long-term strategies to complement the dynamic nature of dementia. This includes the autonomous selection of appropriate prompts to match the user's abilities and current context, using prompts that range from simplistic (e.g., an audio prompt that says "Turn the water

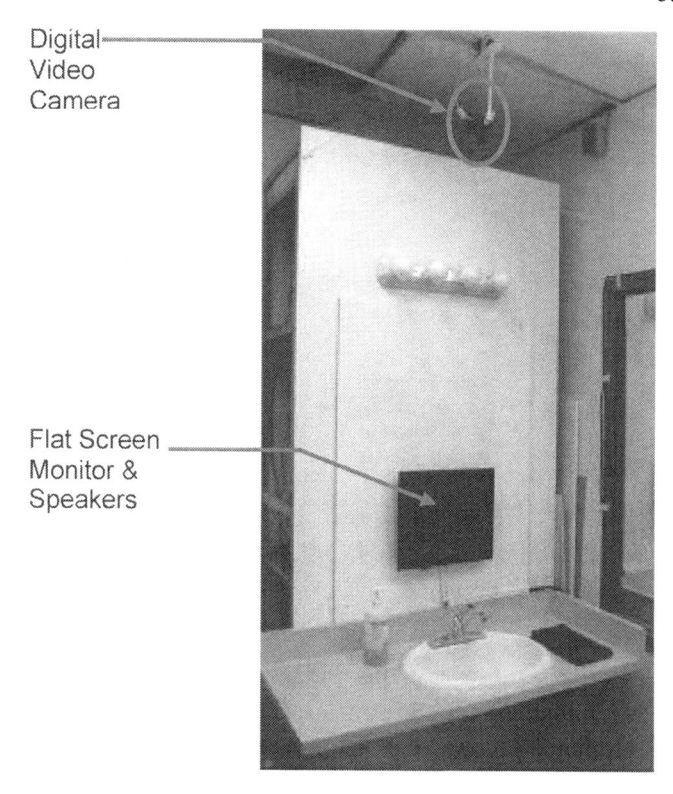

Figure 5.2: The components that make up an installed version of COACH—a webcam overhead to provide input to the system, and a flat screen monitor with speakers to display the necessary prompts.

on") to specific (e.g., an audio prompt "John, push the silver handle to turn the water on" with an accompanying demonstrative video).

In pilot trials with COACH participants with moderate to severe dementia were significantly more independent, requiring little or no human assistance. Participants with moderate-level dementia were able to complete an average of 11% more handwashing steps independently and required 60% fewer interactions with a human caregiver when COACH was in use. Four of the participants achieved complete or very close to complete independence [71]. Improvements are being made to the tracking and planning modules of COACH with the intention of deploying the device into people's homes for further evaluation. In addition, the system is currently being developed for other ADLs, including toothbrushing, nutrition, and work-related tasks.

COACH is also being adapted and applied to other user populations, such as children with autism. The system uses similar algorithms and approaches as the older adult version with respect to the tracking and decision making algorithms. However, children with autism have very different

56 5. EXAMPLES OF ZETS

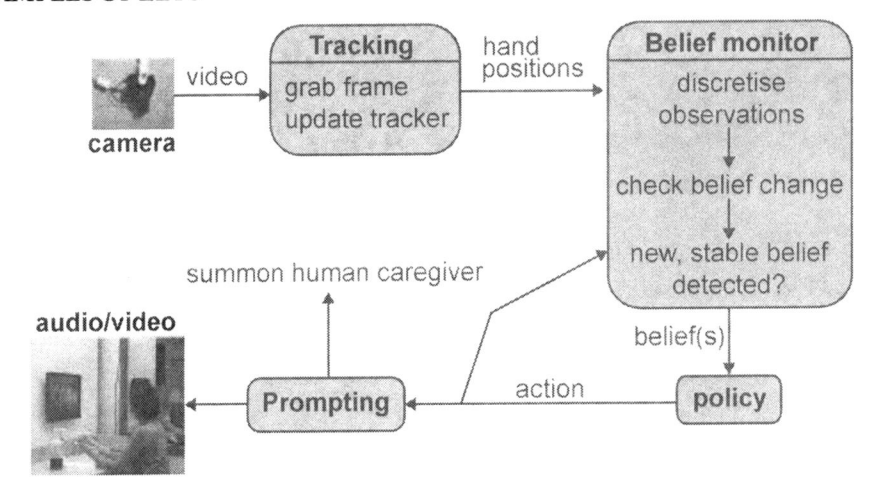

Figure 5.3: The overall architecture for the COACH system, which consists of the tracking, planning (belief monitor and policy), and prompting module.

abilities and mannerisms from older adults with dementia. For instance, while older adults with dementia generally cannot, or do not want to, explicitly interact with a device, most children (with and without autism) enjoy using computerised devices. Also, while caregivers of older adults are often older adults themselves, most do not want to be involved with the technology if it can be avoided. Parents of children with autism, on the other hand, are significantly more eager to understand the technology and want to be able to take an active role in its implementation. Finally, and perhaps most importantly, the nature of the different user types demands different styles of intervention. Dementia results in users requiring devices that should support progressive losses in abilities, while children with autism can and do learn, albeit at a different rate and way than children without autism. Thus, a COACH system for children with autism is designed more as a teaching tool rather than as a compensatory tool, as it is for older adults with dementia.

The primary differences in COACH when it is used with children with autism are that more control is given to caregivers (e.g., parents) to set-up and customize the system for their respective child and that it is possible for the child to explicitly interact with the system. The caregiver is able to change the order and types of audio and visual prompts used, the timing between prompts, and when a caregiver should be called for assistance. Since the system has been designed for children, it possesses features that make the task appear more like a game, including a panel of interactive illuminating push buttons. A child can use the buttons to select rewards and to signal when they think they have completed a step in the task, both of which can be enabled/disabled and customised by a parent. Picture schedules are often used by caregivers to teach ADL and other tasks to children with autism. Picture schedules use a picture to represent each step in a task and markers can be placed to indicate when a step has been completed to help the child keep track of where he or she is in the task. As shown in Figure 5.4, the COACH for autism makes use of an automated picture schedule to indicate progress through the task and the current step the child is on in a way that is familiar to the child.

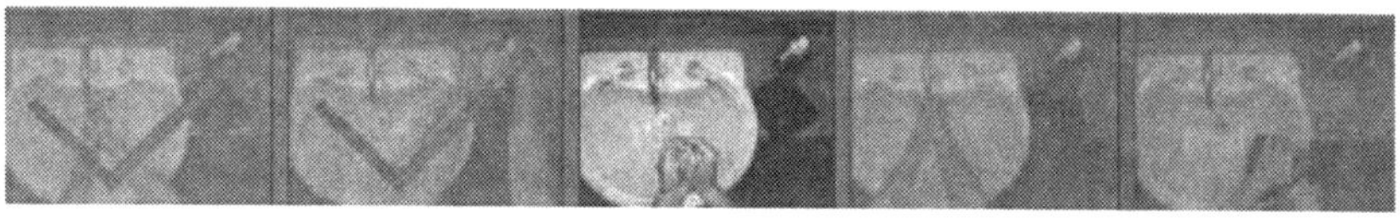

Figure 5.4: Picture schedule for the hand washing task: As the child completes each step, the picture associated with that step is checked off. In this example the child has wet their hands and put soap on their hands, but still needs to scrub, rinse and dry their hands.

5.5 ARCHIPEL

Archipel assists people with cognitive impairments to perform complex "ill-defined" activities of daily living, such as meal preparation, by combining both monitoring (like COACH) with recognition (through RFID and other simple environmental sensors, like Autominder) in a single system [72, 73]. The monitoring module of Archipel analyses errors, feeding this information to the assistance module, which weighs that information against prior experience. Errors are analysed and identified as the user having trouble with initiation, planning, attention, or memory and assistance strategies are employed by Archipel to compensate appropriately.

To begin the process, the user specifies a pre-determined activity using a touchscreen, as shown in Figure 5.5. Monitoring is accomplished as a fusion of explicit (via the touchscreen) and implicit (via RFID-sensor systems) inputs. Guidance can be given to a user via the touchscreen or via indicators mounted in the kitchen, such as LED lights that can highlight items of interest. The system uses a hierarchical planning approach to determine the type of assistance that needs to be provided. Archipel models a task, in this case cooking, according to the different steps that need to be completed and the associated tasks those steps correspond with. Any constraints that need to be adhered to, such as prerequisite steps that need to be completed, etc. are incorporated into this model [72, 73].

Archipel has been tested on 12 cognitively impaired individuals. Preliminary results are positive, indicating a decrease in the number of cues given by the researcher (who plays the role of an assistant or caregiver) when the system is functioning. All participants were able to complete a recipe with Archipel and the overall amount of human assistance was cut in half [72, 73].

As with Autominder and COACH, the developers of Archipel have carefully considered the abilities and needs of the intended user group they are designing for, using inputs, interaction modalities, and types of prompts that work best for this population. Archipel is also designed to

58 5. EXAMPLES OF ZETS

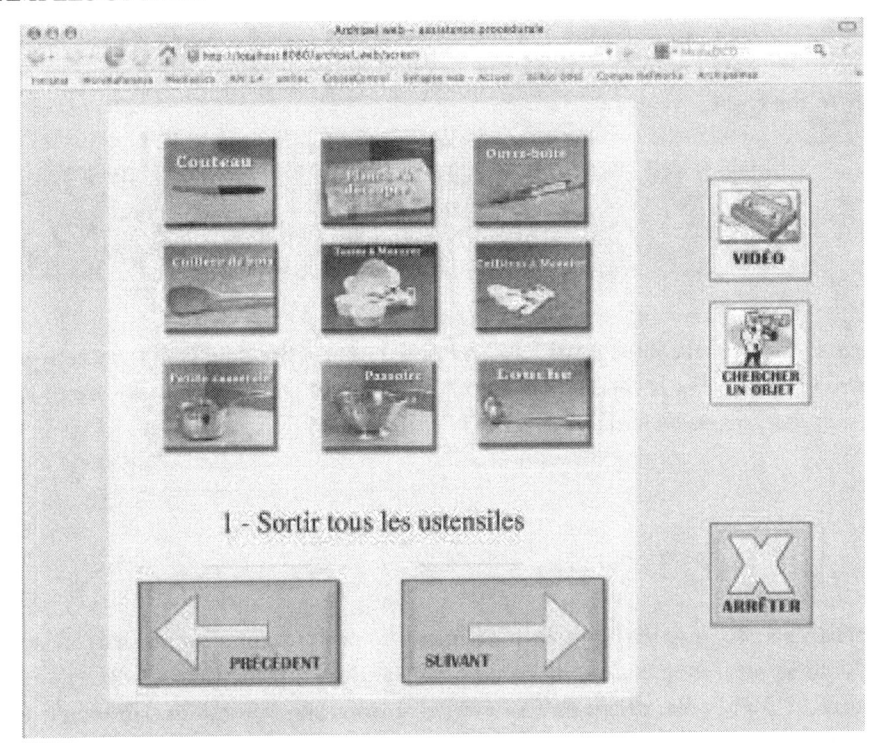

Figure 5.5: The main touchscreen user interface for Archipel, which allows a user to select the required activity.

prompt on an "as-needed" basis, encouraging the user to do as much as he or she can independently of the ZET.

5.6 ASSISTED COGNITION PROJECT

At the mild stages of cognitive impairment, people are often able to still function independently outside of the home, but may easily forget their destination, how to get there, or why they were going there. The Assisted Cognition project [74] was initiated to explore the use of ZETs as a tool to increase the independence and quality of life of older adults with mild Alzheimer's disease.

One of the first devices developed as part of the project was the Activity Compass [75], a tool designed to help disoriented people find their destination. The device consists of a handheld user interface that gives simple directions using a digital arrow similar to a traditional compass. Using a server-based AI engine, destinations are learned automatically based on repetition and duration in particular locations; the system learns the probabilities of where the person is likely to go next based on where they are. This is accomplished by applying Bayes filters to sensor data (e.g., GPS) and determining particular behaviors using state-based Bayesian approaches for modeling and recognition. Based on the where the person most likely wants to go, the handheld device communicates adjusts the direction of the compass arrow accordingly. In this fashion, the Activity Compass autonomously directs a user without him or her having to explicitly input a destination. An extension of the Activity Compass project is Opportunity Knocks, which provided more functionality to the system and expanded its potential user population. Opportunity Knocks [76] is a system designed to provide directional guidance to a cognitive-impaired user navigating through a city. The system infers a user's activities using GPS sensor readings and a hierarchical Markov model. Movement patterns, based on the GPS localization signals, are translated into a probabilistic model using unsupervised learning. From the model and the user's current location, the device is able to predict likely future destinations as well as the associated mode of transportation. Based on the prediction, the system has the ability to prompt the user if an error in route is detected. The user's activities are estimated using a three level dynamic Bayesian network model. The lowest level estimates the user's location, velocity, and mode of transportation from raw GPS sensor readings. The sensor readings are forced to the nearest street on the overall map, providing the user's location. Velocity is determined based on a comparison to the previous location and the amount of time between samples. The mode of transportation is then determined based on the user's velocity. The location of the user's car is tracked, providing differentiation between BUS and CAR, and BUILDING is a mode assigned when the GPS signal is lost beyond a threshold period of time. The second level of the network represents the user's current trip segment and predicted destination. Trip segments are simply defined by a start and end location, and a mode of transportation. The expected route is determined at each intersection the user encounters based on the probability that the user will change direction. Goals are simply the target location of the user. The highest level of the model is a Boolean variable representing whether the system believes it knows the users intention or whether the user is doing something new. If the user is on a known path the system employs the second layer of the model to monitor the user and offers assistance if required. When the user's activities are unknown, the top two levels of the model are removed, the parameters of the lowest level are set to default values and the system monitors the user. Figure 5.6. shows the handheld device and user interface.

5.7 PEAT

PEAT (Planning and Execution Assistant and Trainer) is a ZET that runs on a cell phone and helps compensate for executive function impairment (i.e., the inability to remember sequence of events or tasks), such as users with traumatic brain injury. Similar to the Autominder, PEAT provides assistance by maintaining a schedule of a user's activities and automatically cueing the user when activities need to be started, resumed, or completed. A key aspect of PEAT is the use of reactive planning to adjust a user's schedule when an activity takes an unexpected amount of time to complete, or the user manually updates the calendar [77, 78]. PEAT represents each activity entered by the user as a task, each of which has temporal attributes such as a start time, end time, and expected duration. As the user progresses through their day and updates the status of tasks, PEAT reactively

60   5. EXAMPLES OF ZETS

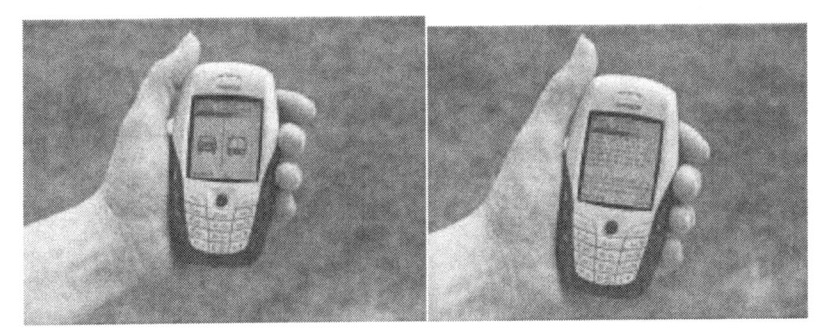

Figure 5.6: A handheld device that automatically determines the mode of transportation, and then gives the user dynamically changing directions to a specific destination.

updates the day's schedule, and advises the user when tasks should start or stop, when conflicts arise, or when decisions must be made. Figure 5.7 shows an example of the PEAT interface and how it prompts a user for a current task.

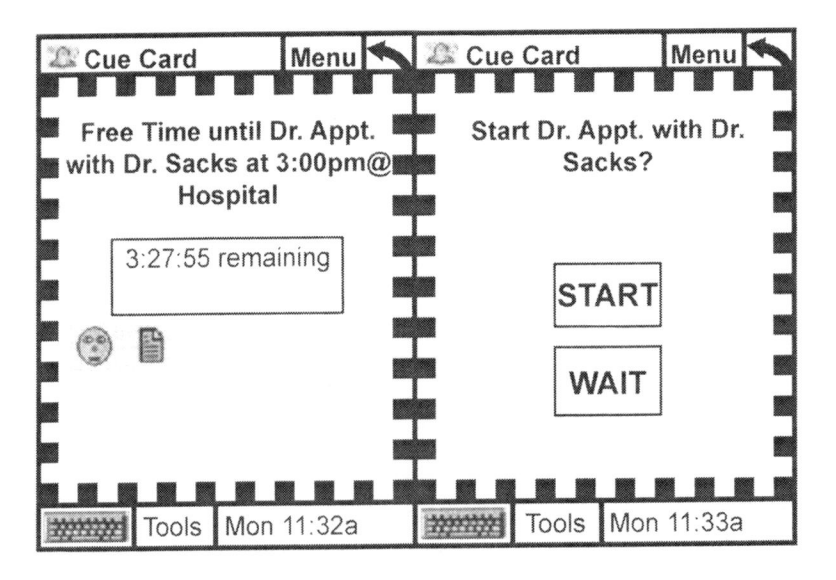

Figure 5.7: To help users stay on task, PEAT uses a unique cue card display to present information about only the current activity, providing reminder cues to start and stop scheduled and scripted activities (From www.brainaid.com).

PEAT uses both planning and activity recognition algorithms to schedule (or re schedule) activities as necessary. With respect to the planning algorithms, PEAT uses an AI planning system called PROPEL (PROgram Planning and Execution Language) [77]. In PROPEL, users develop scripts for routine tasks such as activities required in the morning or going out shopping for groceries. The most important feature of PROPEL is that the same script can be used for both planning and execution. Planning involves simulating the script before it is executed. Scripts can contain choice points that identify where a choice must be selected from a set of alternative resources or subroutines. Examples of choice points in a "Dinner" script include choosing a restaurant for dinner and choosing between walking or driving. Without any planning a default script can be executed reactively by using heuristics to make default choice point selections. The planner first simulates the default program instance, and then simulates program variations. The planner evaluates each simulation with respect to the goals, and it searches for program variations that maximize goal achievement. Finally, the planner generates advice rules that are used during execution to make deliberate selections at choice points [77].

5.8 PROACT

The PROACT system is an example of a ZET that uses machine learning for the specific purpose of inferring the tasks being completed based on sensor inputs. This system has three components: body worn RFID sensors (as shown in Figure 5.8), a probabilistic engine that infers activities given observations from these sensors, and a model creator that easily creates probabilistic models of activities [79].

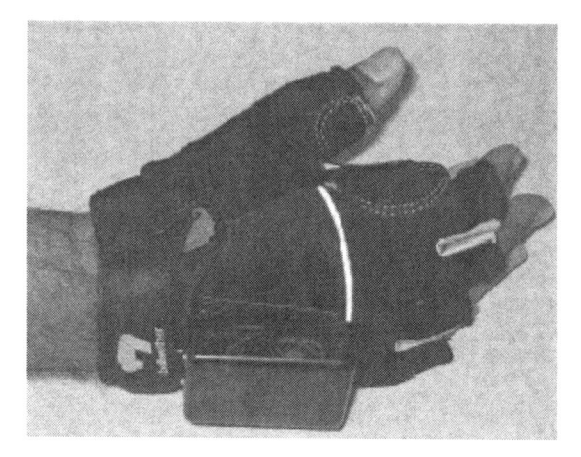

Figure 5.8: The PROACT system used on-person RFID tags in the form of a glove that would then detect which objects the person was interacting with in the environment (From [79]).

PROACT uses a dynamic Bayesian network (DBN) to infer activities that represents daily activities such as making tea, washing, and brushing teeth. Each activity type that PROACT is intended to recognize is modeled as a linear series of steps, where specific objects that are involved in the completion of each step and the probability of seeing each such object are assigned. For example, making tea is modeled as three different steps, in which there is high probability of using the tea kettle in the first step, a high probability of using the box of tea bags in the second step, and medium probability of using milk, sugar, or lemon in the third step [79]. The probabilities are able to capture three possible sources of error: sensor noise, unknown objects in the model, and optional objects used in each step. The probabilistic engine converts these activity models into a set of dynamic Bayesian networks (DBN). The current sub-activity is modeled as a hidden variable in the DBN (as this is not explicitly known) and the set of objects seen and the time elapsed are modeled as observed variables (as these can be empirically determined). Bayesian filtering can be used to estimate the activities from sensor data. As the DBNs grow quite large, PROACT is required to use a sequential Monte Carlo approximation to solve for the most likely activities. Using the full DBN rather than a simpler HMM-based model allows the system to handle partially ordered activities and an explicit model of time (both of which are elements that drastically expand the size of the DBN) [79].

Recent work in the same direction has investigated how activities can be modeled with a combination of discriminative and generative approaches [80], how common sense models of everyday activities can be built automatically using data mining techniques [38, 81], and how human activities can be analyzed through the recognition of object use, rather than the recognition of human behavior [82]. The last work uses DBNs as well to model various activities around the home, and a variety of radio frequency identification (RFID) tags to bootstrap the learning process.

5.9 EPAD

Being able to express oneself and participate in leisure activities is crucial to maintaining one's identity, reducing stress, and communicating with others. Older adults with dementia often have trouble with social-based tasks, particularly those that rely on executive memory functioning, which can lead to feelings of isolation and depression. The ePAD is an example of a ZET that has been designed to promote participation in leisure activities, specifically engaging older adults with dementia in creative arts tasks. This ZET was developed to mimic a typical art easel, as this type of interface is familiar to older adults, particularly if they are already engaging in art therapy. As shown in Figure 5.9, the user interface (a painting program in this case) is displayed on the device's canvas, which is touch sensitive and can handle multiple touch inputs at a time [83]. ePAD can be configured by an arts therapist or caregiver to have tools (e.g., virtual paint brushes, stamps, images, etc.) or themes that they feel the person interacting with the device would enjoy using, enabling the tools and canvas background to be personalised to each user.

A webcam is used to observe the user's face and computer vision algorithms are used to identify whether someone is looking at the screen. Information about where the user is looking and their interaction with the screen (e.g., where they have been touching) are passed to the AI system, which uses a partially observable Markov decision process (POMDP) model to estimate the person's current state (i.e., what they are currently doing). The POMDP model accomplishes this by using prior information about what inputs it is most likely to see as a result of different actions by the user

5.9. EPAD

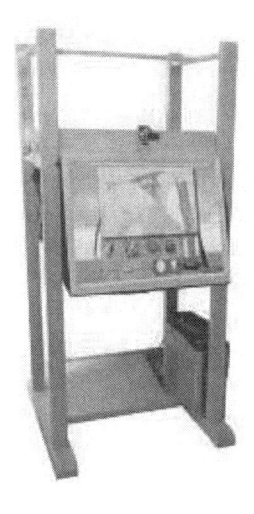

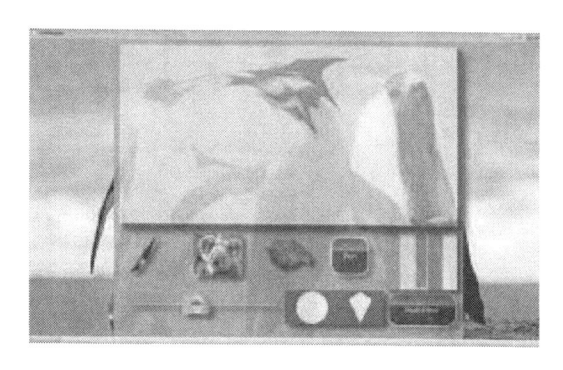

Figure 5.9: The ePAD was developed to look like a typical art easel, with a multi-touch screen in place of a canvas to allow the user to perform different painting activities.

to deduce what is likely going on based on incoming observations (data). For example, the POMDP knows that a person who is *engaged* with the device will often spend more time with his/her finger on the screen. Therefore, if a user keeps his/her finger on the screen (an observation) longer, the POMDP will interpret this as the user being more engaged. The device is also able to estimate how responsive the person is to certain prompts, what level of behavioural activation he/she is exhibiting (e.g., are they being very active or are they inactive), and what elements of the application he/she has used or completed (e.g., if the screen is full of colour). Based on these observations and estimates, the device selects an action to take that is appropriate for what the user is doing and what his/her preferences are, such as highlighting different tools the user could try. This action is delivered to the canvas and can be accompanied by an audio prompt [83]. Importantly, the system actions and the interface itself are all full programmable by art therapists. This ZET explicitly incorporates this secondary user (as previously defined in Section 3.1.2 on User-Centred Design), giving him or her the ability to be involved in the design of the device for a particular client. The overall system architecture is shown in Figure 5.10.

The ZET was designed using many of the techniques and design criteria described in this lecture, including an intensively user-centred design approach through a participatory design methodology. Through an online questionnaire and multiple focus groups with the researchers, art therapists participated in the design of the system, including the functions, features, and layout of the user interface. In addition to the physical characteristics of the device, topics that were discussed included the identification of contextual factors that are important in this particular activity, as well as the outcomes and goals that one might want to achieve [83].

64   5. EXAMPLES OF ZETS

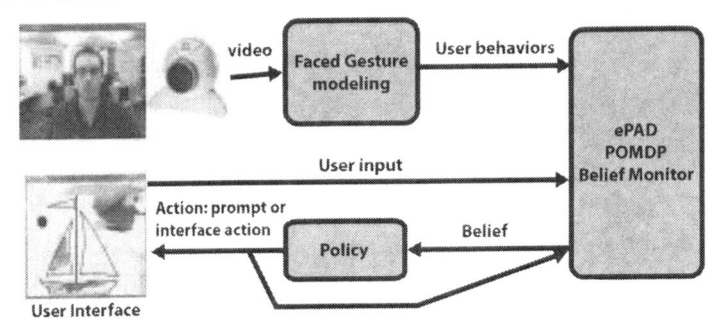

Figure 5.10: The overall ePAD system architecture.

5.10 THE HELPER

The HELPER (Health Evaluation and Logging Personal Emergency Response) system is an example of a ZET that is primarily used to ensure the safety and health of users in a home or institution. Following the ZET paradigm, the HELPER employs AI methods, such as computer vision, machine learning, and speech recognition, to automatically monitor a user in his or her home and detect adverse events, such as a fall, without the need for the user to initiate a call for help. Importantly, the device is very easy to use as it does not require occupants (users) to wear any markers and uses a speech-based interface (i.e., the user and device talk to each other). A complete working prototype that focuses on fall detection has been designed, implemented, tested, and is undergoing iterative design improvements through a series of real-life in-home experiments. As shown in Figure 5.11, the current version of the system is a self-contained device that is installed on the ceiling in any room that requires monitoring.

Computer vision and video analysis techniques are used for background subtraction, tracking the shapes of moving objects (humans, etc.) within the scene and to extract a set of features that correlate with falls. An example of this process is illustrated in Figure 5.12. The incoming video stream is not stored, but rather is analysed by the system in real-time vision before being discarded. Subsequently, machine learning techniques, applied to carefully engineered features, allow the system to identify when a fall has likely occurred. Upon the detection of a fall, the system initiates a conversation with the person to determine the level of emergency, as well as if and what type of assistance they would like. A brief number of "yes/no" questions are asked at this stage and automatic speech recognition is used to determine the user's responses. Typical questions include "Hello Mary, do you need help?", "Do you want me to call an ambulance?", or "Do you want me to call your daughter?" If the victim is unresponsive (e.g., he or she is unconscious or their speech unintelligible), the system defaults into connecting them to a live operator for further investigation. Moreover, as the system is speech-based, it is possible for the user to initialise a call for help even if the system cannot "see" him or her by the user calling out to the system. It is important to note that the only

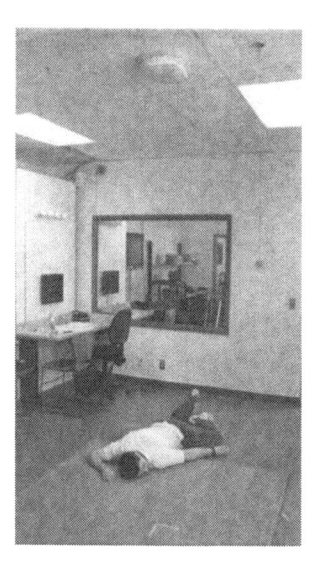

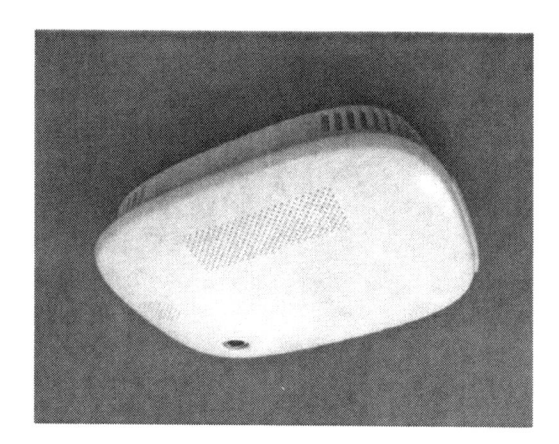

Figure 5.11: The ceiling-mounted HELPER system can autonomously detect falls and then have a dialogue with the occupant to procure appropriate assistance.

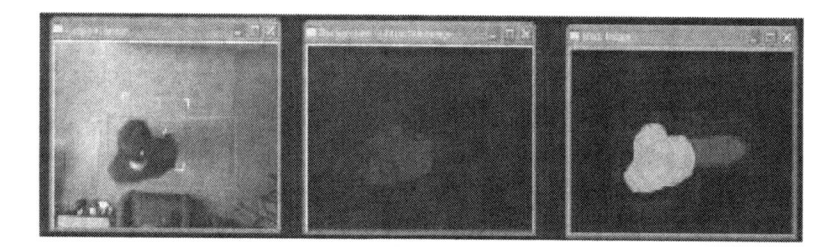

Figure 5.12: Example frames from the overhead unit that illustrates the extraction of a person from the background and then separate analyses on the blob representing the user and his or her shadow.

data that is sent out is the notification of an adverse event and consequential choices of action, which are determined by the user and the system. This approach not only saves on the transmission and storage of large amounts of data but also implicitly protects people's privacy.

The first prototype of the HELPER system [84] used an off-the-shelf webcam, equipped with a microphone, for data collection. It applied various image processing techniques, such as background subtraction and blob analysis to classify the posture of a user. Once the image has been processed, it then used an artificial neural network to classify the posture as a fall or non-fall. Following extensive laboratory testing, the system was tested in two homes of healthy young adults who were instructed to simulate fall events several times daily for a week apiece. After identified deficiencies were corrected following the first trial, the system was able to detect 100% of the simulated falls in the second set of trials. However, approximately five false alarms per day also occurred because of more complex situations than the system had been exposed to up to that point, such as a shadow cast by a tree through a window and novel interactions when multiple occupants were present.

An improved version of the system has subsequently been developed to ameliorate limitations observed during the in-home trials [85]. The improvements include: the use of a wide-angle lens to increase the area of coverage; dealing with the resulting image distortion; enhancing robustness to abrupt lighting changes and lighting effects such as sunlight through a window; and handling more than one subject by tracking multiple foreground regions. These limitations are primarily being solved through the use of more complex machine learning algorithms, such as a support vector machine learning, in order to extract novel features that better differentiate between a fallen person and other occurrences in the image, such as shadows, furniture, and pets.

5.11 REHABILITATION ROBOTICS

ZETs have more recently been incorporated into rehabilitation to help clients complete a variety of different types of exercises and programs, and in particular, to assist with post-stroke rehabilitation. An example of this is the stroke rehabilitation robot that is being developed at the Toronto Rehabilitation Institute. This project in particular is classified as a ZET as it employs an AI controller that enables the robot to make its own decisions with respect to adjusting the parameters of a client's rehabilitation regime. Thus, this system attempts to increase the amount, complexity, and appropriateness of a client's rehabilitation regime while simultaneously reducing the amount of supervision and input required from therapists. Moreover, the device is able to give the client and therapist quantitative data regarding the client's performance, which can be used to motivate the client and inform the therapist of the client's progress.

The rehabilitation stroke robot is currently designed to guide post-stroke clients through an upper-limb rehabilitation reaching task [86]. An upper-limb reaching exercise was selected as upper extremities are typically affected more than the lower extremities after stroke and gross upper-limb motion is the basic motion involved for many activities of daily living, such as getting out of a chair, picking up objects, and getting dressed. The overall system is comprised of a robotic device, virtual environment, and an intelligent system, as illustrated in Figure 5.13. As shown in Figure 5.14, the robotic platform has two degrees of freedom, which allow a reaching exercise to be performed in 2D space by moving the end-effector of the robot. The robotic device also incorporates haptic technology to provide resistance and boundary guidance for the user during the exercise. Encoders in the end-effector of the robotic device provide data to indicate hand position and shoulder abduction/internal rotation during the exercise. The system also includes postural sensors that provide data to indicate trunk rotation compensation (i.e., to ensure that the person using the device is using their arm to reach and not moving their trunk). The virtual system provides visual feedback to the person doing the exercise. The current AI-based planning system is implemented using a partially observable Markov decision process (POMDP) model [87, 88]. In this system, observation data from the robotic device

5.11. REHABILITATION ROBOTICS 67

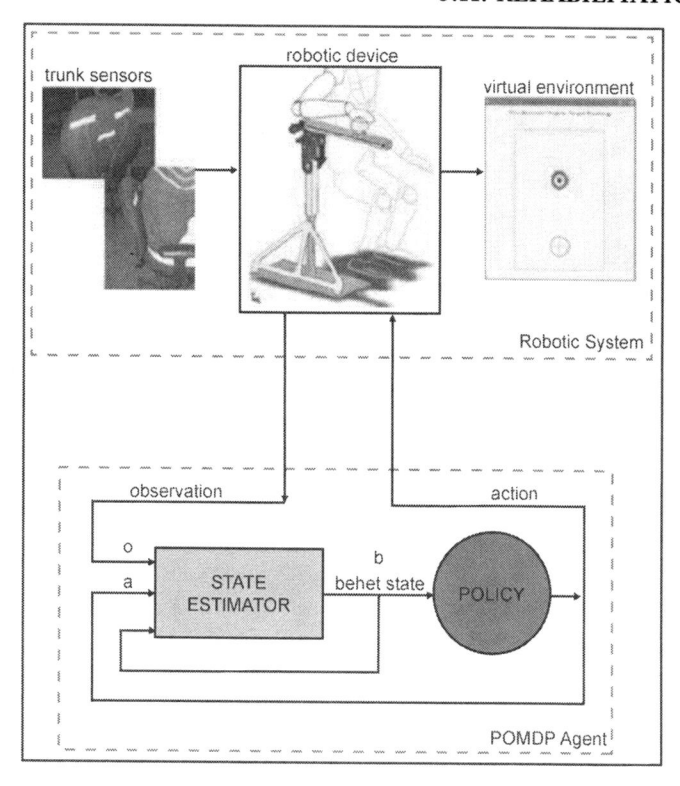

Figure 5.13: The overall robotic system consists of the robot (including various posture sensors), a graphical user interface, and an intelligent system that uses a POMDP model (agent).

are passed to the POMDP model where a state estimator estimates the probable progress of the user. A policy then maps this estimate, or belief state, to an action for the system to execute which can be either setting a new target position, setting a new resistance level, or stopping the exercise. The goal of the POMDP agent is to help clients regain their maximum reaching distance at the most difficult level of resistance, while performing the exercises with control and proper posture. However, the system needs to balance these goals against possible fatigue and strain, to ensure the client is not pushed beyond his or her abilities.

To date, the performance of the robotic stroke device has been evaluated by comparing the decisions made by the system with those of an expert through a study where a single post-stroke participant was paired up with a professional physiotherapist. Overall, the therapist agreed with the system's decisions approximately 65% of the time. In general, the therapist thought the system decisions were credible and could envision this system being used in both a clinical and home setting. The client was satisfied with the system and said that she would use this system as her primary method of rehabilitation.

68 5. EXAMPLES OF ZETS

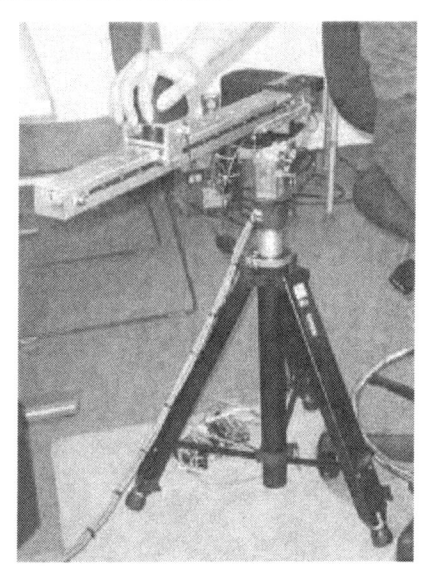

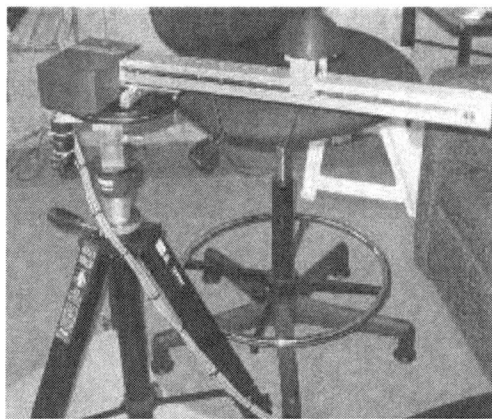

Figure 5.14: The upper-limb stroke robotic rehabilitation device.

A next version of this ZET is currently under development. The research team is applying several of the design principles outlined previously to expand the efficacy, applicability, and capabilities of the device. Specifically, a user-centred approach is being used to discern opinions and needs of therapists and to involve them in the design process. An international online survey with post-stroke rehabilitation therapists was conducted during the spring and summer of 2010 to understand current rehabilitation practices, as well as what robotic rehabilitation device features therapists would be interested in. Using the results of the survey [89], the design team has redesigned the robotic platform and are currently developing virtual games with 2D target locations and a new probabilistic framework, which, similarly to the previous POMDP version, includes online learning capability that adapts to each individual patient's need and produces varying levels of resistance during the exercise. The POMDP model is being further developed by including models of the continuous relationship between the target resistance and the ability of the user to reach each distance [90]. A second type of planning agent is also being developed using a fuzzy logic-based intelligent system that mimics the reasoning of a therapist during the exercise using a set of fuzzy rule bases [91]. Like the POMDP version, the fuzzy system includes both resistive and assistive forces in order to improve user performance during the exercise.

CHAPTER 6

Conclusions and Future Directions

6.1 LIMITATIONS OF ZETS

This lecture has provided an overview of the design, development, and testing of ZETs. It has provided examples of different systems that have been developed and has given evidence that ZET use could have a significant impact on the care of people with disabilities. However, it should be recognized that this field is still in its infancy. While considerable research and development efforts are underway, there are still limitations in this area of work that are preventing ZETs from becoming pervasively available as commercial products.

One limitation is the performance and robustness of the current AI algorithms and sensing hardware. While these fields have progressed tremendously over the past several years, especially with the influx of new hardware platforms and computer processors, significant research still needs to be conducted with new techniques and approaches to ensure resulting systems are dependable and appropriate. For example, computer vision is becoming a more popular sensing modality in ZETs, however, many of the techniques being used are not robust enough to deal with real-world contexts and environments, such as changing lighting conditions within a room and multiple occupants in a house.

Another limitation is the lack of clinical data and real-world evidence that ZETs can have a significant effect on the health and wellness of people with disabilities. While there have been many different technologies developed, many of these have only been tested in limited user trials that often include only a small sample of subjects, who are more often than not, not real users. Usability and efficacy studies with ZETs tend to be conducted in simulated environments with simulated users, such as healthy adults or actors who attempt to portray the targeted user impairments. It is extremely rare in the literature to find in-depth, long-term trials, such as randomized controlled trials (RCT). As such, when compared with research studies in other healthcare fields, the strength of evidence for the use of ZETs is relatively low. However, much of this is a result of the newness of the field, namely, that the technologies under development are just reaching the stages where they are ready to be tried in real-world deployments for long periods of time. As the field matures and devices become more robust, more clinical trials will emerge.

This lecture also provided an overview of key design paradigms and approaches that can be used in the development of ZETs. However, a limitation in this process is that a common framework, or guideline, does not currently exist for designers and researchers to follow. As a result, the ZET field has become somewhat fragmented with different types of devices being developed that are not compatible, cannot be easily used together, and do not have efficacy outcomes that can be assessed and compared. While the principles of pervasive computing are often discussed in this field, it is very rare that they are adhered to. This is not only true with respect to ZETs under development, but also for ZETs and assistive technologies that are currently commercially available. For example, as previously described, there is significant research being conducted on intelligent systems for powered wheelchairs, such as anti-collision and navigation systems. However, the majority of these devices are only compatible with the powered wheelchair that they were originally developed for and would require significant modifications to work with different chairs. A common framework that provided design criteria with respect to issues surrounding such topics as communication protocols and other pervasive computing principles would alleviate many of these compatibility limitations.

Finally, there are current "practical" limitations with current ZETs, namely issues around device installation and operation. As many of these new devices are being developed to be completely embedded into their environments, installation is becoming a significant challenge especially when many different sensors and computing units need to be mounted on ceilings, walls, etc. For example, the fall detection system that was previously described needs to be installed on the ceiling of each room that requires monitoring. These types of installations become even more difficult when retrofitting spaces that may not be conducive to supporting these technologies, such as an older home. Related to installation is also the need to power these new devices and systems. As many current ZETs require advanced processing and computing systems to operate, these devices cannot simply use batteries; they have power needs that require being hardwired or "plugged in" to a power source. Using the fall detection system as an example once again, a limiting factor in the adoption of this type of technology may be the fact that each ceiling mounted unit requires a power connection in the ceiling, or power cables to be run to the nearest outlet. While potential solutions exist, such as retrofitting a ceiling light fixture with the ZET, many potential consumers of ZETs may not have this type of infrastructure available in their homes, nor would they want to run cables along ceilings and walls. A potential operational limitation is that all of these new systems rely on current infrastructures, such as computer networks, already being in place and working. If, for example, the computer network that is used for the different system components to communicate with each other failed, then the entire system would fail as well. As such, more robust computer and data networks need to be developed to make ZETs more reliable and robust.

6.2 FUTURE CHALLENGES AND CONSIDERATIONS

Despite their current limitations, the future of ZETs is promising and will very likely continue to become more important as the population grows older and the number of people who have some kind of disability or impairment increases. As described in this lecture, in order to be effective these technologies need to be easily adaptable to these users' needs. The requirement for this adaptability to be automatically performed by the technology will become even more important as the trend towards providing care to people with disabilities in their own homes becomes more prevalent.

The ability to age in place, at any age, is a win-win situation as this enables the person to choose where they wish to reside and care administered in a non-institutional setting can ease pressures on formal healthcare systems, particularly if it is augmented by assistive technology. In response, advanced sensing, machine learning, and other applications from the fields of pervasive computing and artificial intelligence will continue to play a large role in the development of future ZETs. This will be true not only for those technologies related to cognition, but also to those needed for mobility and sensory impairments. It is becoming apparent that ZETs can no longer just focus on the single dimension of cognition, but must also take into account the other co-morbidities that users may face. For example, there is growing literature in the area of intelligent powered wheelchairs that can help people with cognitive impairments navigate their environments more safely [92, 93]. There has also been work to add intelligence and complex sensing to more "traditional" assistive technologies such as walkers and canes to help users to maintain their balance and to help with wayfinding. In addition, there are several new frontiers that are starting to be explored that can have a significant impact on the lives of people with disabilities. One potential area is the use of advanced robotics to help care for users with a variety of disabilities. For example, it could be imagined that personal robotics can play a significant role in supporting people who require care in their own homes. Robots can be developed that can help complete a variety of activities, such as meal preparation or house work, and could also play a role in the monitoring and assessment of a person's overall health and well-being. Within the area of ZETs to help monitor the health and well-being of people with disabilities, researchers are developing ways of placing sensors into building materials. Dubbed *brick computing*, this approach creates pervasive computing systems that are made out of building materials themselves. Embedding a variety of sensors into floor, wall, and ceiling materials allows for continuous and autonomous ambient readings, without any kind of manual interactions from the user. Researchers at the University of Toronto are developing a floor tile that will be able to measure a person's physiological parameters (e.g., heart rate and blood pressure) simply by the person standing on the tile in bare feet. This way, a person's physiological data could be captured several times a day in a home environment, allowing for a much richer, long-term picture of the person's health, which could be used to help inform treatment options and help people understand and actively manage their own health.

The future of ZETs demands more work to be completed on the development and use of new design paradigms that will allow for data to be collected with respect to user needs. While traditional approaches, such as user-centred design, are proving to be useful, it is still difficult to include this population in the design process. This is especially true with vulnerable or frail users, such as older adults with dementia or other cognitive impairments. The dynamic nature of disabilities is forcing this field to begin to incorporate design and evaluation strategies that are as equally dynamic. However, issues around how to incorporate these new approaches while still being able to construct prototypes effectively, in a timely manner, and without increasing the end costs of the resulting technology, are still significant barriers that need to be addressed.

6. CONCLUSIONS AND FUTURE DIRECTIONS

As ZETs become more ubiquitous in healthcare institutions, communities, and homes, more research on the social and ethical implications of these types of technologies needs to be conducted. In particular, special considerations need to be taken in the design and use of these technologies when the targeted user is unable to make an informed decision or consent about the ZET's use, such as people with cognitive disabilities and children. This issue becomes even more problematic as more ZETs are developed for private and personal activities and are installed in sensitive locations (e.g., in the bathroom). Careful consideration needs to be taken in determining how consent will be obtained to use these new technologies, and how users will be educated about the potential benefits and limitations of these systems in a fashion that is consistent with their cognitive abilities. These issues have not been fully addressed within this field of technologies and hold the potential for a new and fruitful area of research.

In conclusion, while ZETs are still in their infancy and are not yet commercially available, they demonstrate tremendous potential in their ability to provide customised and dynamic support with little or no effort on the part of the primary user or their caregiver. Moreover, the rich and continuous data collected by ZETs could enable clinicians and others in a person's circle of care to make more informed decisions regarding interventions, which could, in turn, significantly improve a person's well being. The nature of ZETs also means that they must be carefully designed and tested, as a misuse of data or an error on the part of the ZET could have serious consequences. As such, ZETs must be developed in a way that always holds the end users' well-being as the paramount goal and includes the stakeholders in the design process from start to finish ensuring the resulting technologies are appropriate, useful, and accepted.

References

[1] World Health Organization, "Towards a Common Language for Functioning, Disability and Health: ICF," World Health Organization, Geneva, Switzerland 2002. Cited on page(s) 5, 37

[2] G. Abowd, M. Ebling, G. Hung, H. Lei, and H. W. Gellerson, "Context-aware Computing," *Pervasive Computing*, vol. July-September, pp. 22–23, 2002. Cited on page(s) 6

[3] J. E. Bardram, "Applications of context-aware computng in hospital work: Examples and design principles," in *ACM Symposium on Applied Computing*, Nicosia, Cyprus, 2004, pp. 1574–1579. DOI: 10.1145/967900.968215 Cited on page(s) 6

[4] A. Dey, "Understanding and Using Context," *Journal of Personal and Ubiquitous Computing*, vol. 5, pp. 4–7, 2001. DOI: 10.1007/s007790170019 Cited on page(s)

[5] D. Salber, A. Dey, and G. Abowd, "The context toolkit: Aiding the development of context-enabled applications," in *Conference on Human Factors in Computing Systems (CHI)*, 1999. DOI: 10.1145/302979.303126 Cited on page(s) 24

[6] B. Schilit, N. Adams, and R. Want, "Context-aware computing application," in *The First Workshop on Mobile Computing Systems and Applications*, Santa Cruz, CA, 1994, pp. 85–90. DOI: 10.1109/WMCSA.1994.16 Cited on page(s) 6

[7] J. E. Bardram, A. Mihailidis, and D. Wan, *Pervasive Computing in Healthcare*. Boca Raton, FL: CRC Press, 2007. Cited on page(s) 6, 9

[8] J. Paradiso, "Guest Editors' Introduction: Smart Energy Systems," *IEEE Pervasive Computing* vol. January, pp. 11–12, 2011. DOI: 10.1109/MPRV.2011.4 Cited on page(s) 6

[9] (2011, August 6, 2011). *Smart grid conceptual framework diagram*. Available: http://smartgrid.ieee.org/smart-grid-framework-diagram Cited on page(s) 6, 7, 8

[10] U. Hansmann, L. Merk, M. S. Nicklous, and T. Stober, "Chapter 1: What Pervasive Computing is all About," in *Pervasive Computing, 2nd Edition*, Spring, Ed., ed New York: Spring-Verlag, 2003, pp. 11–22. Cited on page(s) 6, 7, 8, 10, 12

[11] G. W. Arnold, "Challenges and opportunities in smart grid: A position articile," *Proceedings of the IEEE*, vol. 99, pp. 922–927, 2011. DOI: 10.1109/JPROC.2011.2125930 Cited on page(s) 7

74 REFERENCES

[12] V. Sundramoorthy, "Domesticating energy-monitoring systems: Challenges and design concers," *IEEE Pervasive Computing,* vol. 1, pp. 20–27, 2011. DOI: 10.1109/MPRV.2010.73 Cited on page(s) 8, 9

[13] D. Bergman, "Nonintrusive load-shed verification," *IEEE Pervasive Computing,* vol. 1, pp. 49–57, 2011. DOI: 10.1109/MPRV.2010.71 Cited on page(s) 8

[14] Department of Commerce. (2011, August 6, 2011). *NIST & The Smart Grid.* Available: http://www.nist.gov/smartgrid/nistandsmartgrid.cfm Cited on page(s) 9, 10

[15] M. Pollack and B. Peintner, "Computer science tools and techniques," in *Pervasive Computing in Healthcare,* J. E. Bardram, A. Mihailidis, and D. Wan, Eds., ed Boca Raton, FL: CRC Press, 2007, pp. 21–40. Cited on page(s) 9, 10, 11, 12

[16] A. Cavoukian, "Privacy by Design: The 7 foundational principle," Information & Privacy Commissioner of Ontario, Toronto 2011. Cited on page(s) 12, 33

[17] L. Chen, C. Nugent, J. Biswas, and J. Hoey, *Activity Recognition in Pervasive Intelligent Environments.* London, UK: Atlantis Press, 2011. Cited on page(s) 13, 24

[18] R. Szeliski, *Computer Vision: Algorithms and Applications.* New York, NY: Springer, 2010. Cited on page(s) 13, 16

[19] G. Bradski and A. Kaehler, *Learning OpenCV*: O'Reilly Media, 2008. Cited on page(s) 13, 16

[20] R. Want, *RFID Explained: A Primer on Radio Frequency Identification Technologies*: Morgan & Claypool Publishers, 2006. Cited on page(s) 15

[21] L. Shapiro and G. Stockman, *Computer Vision*: Prentice Hall, 2001. Cited on page(s) 16

[22] D. Forsyth and J. Ponce, *Computer Vision: A Modern Approach.* Upper Saddle River, NJ: Prentice Hall, 2002. Cited on page(s) 16

[23] R. O. Duda and P. E. Hart, *Pattern Classification and Scene Analysis*: John Wiley and Sons, 2002. Cited on page(s) 16, 17, 19

[24] C. M. Bishop, *Pattern Recognition and Machine Learning*: Springer, 2006. Cited on page(s) 16, 17, 18, 19, 23, 24

[25] D. J. C. MacKay, *Information Theory, Inference, and Learning Algorithms*: Cambridge University Press, 2003. Cited on page(s) 17, 22, 23, 26

[26] C. Rasmussen, "Joint Likelihood Methods for Mitigating Visual Tracking Disturbances," presented at the Proceedings of the IEEE Workshop on Multi-Object Tracking, 2001. DOI: 10.1109/MOT.2001.937983 Cited on page(s)

REFERENCES 75

[27] R. Sutton and A. G. Barto, *Reinforcement Learning: An Introduction*: MIT Press, 1998. Cited on page(s) 17, 20

[28] D. Poole and A. Mackworth, *Artificial Intelligence: Foundations of Computational Agents*. Cambridge, UK: Cambridge University Press, 2010. Cited on page(s) 17

[29] S. Russell and P. Norvig, *Artificial Intelligence: A Modern Approach*. New Jersey: Prentice Hall, 1995. Cited on page(s) 17, 18

[30] J. R. Quinlan, *C4.5: Programs for Machine Learning*. San Mateo, CA: Morgan Kaufmann, 1993. Cited on page(s) 18

[31] M. Markou and S. Singh, "Novelty detection: A review - part 1: Statistical approaches," *Signal Processing*, vol. 83, p. 2003, 2003. DOI: 10.1016/j.sigpro.2003.07.018 Cited on page(s) 19

[32] C.-H. Teh and R. T. Chin, "On Image Analysis by the Methods of Moments," *IEEE Transactions on Pattern Analysis and Machine Intelligence*, vol. 10, pp. 496–513, July 1988. DOI: 10.1109/34.3913 Cited on page(s) 19

[33] T. Kohonen, *Self-Organization and Associative Memory*. Berlin: Springer-Verlag, 1989. Cited on page(s) 19

[34] D. Koller and N. Friedman, *Probabilistic Graphical Models: Principles and Techniques*. Cambridge, MA: MIT Press, 2009. Cited on page(s) 20, 22, 23

[35] R. Bellman, *Dynamic Programming*. Princeton, NJ: Princeton University Press, 1957. Cited on page(s) 20

[36] M. L. Puterman, *Markov Decision Processes: Discrete Stochastic Dynamic Programming*. New York, NY.: Wiley, 1994. Cited on page(s) 20

[37] M. O. Duff, "Optimal Learning: Computational procedures for Bayes-adaptive Markov decision processes," University of Massassachusetts Amherst, 2002. Cited on page(s) 21

[38] W. Pentney, M. Philipose, and J. Bilmes, "Structure learning on large scale common sense statistical models of human state," presented at the Proc. AAAI, Chicago, 2008. Cited on page(s) 24, 62

[39] L. Chen, C. Nugent, M. Mulvenna, D. Finlay, X. Hong, and M. Poland, "A logical framework for behaviour reasoning and assistance in a smart home," *International Journal of Assistive Robotics and Mechatronics*, vol. 9, p. 2034, 2008. Cited on page(s) 24

[40] F. Mastrogiovanni, A. Sgorbissa, and R. Zaccaria, "An integrated approach to context specification and recognition in smart homes," in *Smart Homes and Health Telematics*, 2008, p. 2633. DOI: 10.1007/978-3-540-69916-3_4 Cited on page(s) 24

REFERENCES

[41] J. Hoey, T. Ploetz, D. Jackson, P. Olivier, A. F. Monk, and C. Pham, "Rapid specification and automated generation of prompting systems to assist with people with dementia," in *Pervasive and Mobile Computing*, 2011. DOI: 10.1016/j.pmcj.2010.11.007 Cited on page(s) 25

[42] H. Ryu and A. F. Monk, "Interaction Unit Analysis: A new interaction design framework," *HCI*, 2009. DOI: 10.1080/07370020903038086 Cited on page(s) 25

[43] L. Chen and P. Pu, "A survey of preference elicitation methods," EPFL2004. Cited on page(s) 25

[44] M. Follette Story, "Maximizing Usability: The Principle of Universal Design," *Assistive Technology*, vol. 10, pp. 4–12, 1998. DOI: 10.1080/10400435.1998.10131955 Cited on page(s) 28

[45] D. A. Norman, *The Design of Everyday Things*. New York: Basic Books, 2002. Cited on page(s) 30

[46] J. D. Gould and C. Lewis, "Designing for usability: Key principles and what designers think," *Communications of ACM*, vol. 28, pp. 300–311, 1985. DOI: 10.1145/3166.3170 Cited on page(s) 30

[47] C. Wickens, *Engineering Psychology and Human Performance*, 2nd ed. New York: Harper Collins Publishers, 1992. Cited on page(s) 30

[48] J. Preece, Y. Rogers, and H. Sharp, *Interaction Design*. Wiley & Sons, 2002. Cited on page(s) 31

[49] T. Adlam, R. Orpwood, and T. Dunn, "User evaluation in pervasive healthcare," in *Pervasive Computing in Healthcare*, J. E. Bardram, A. Mihailidis, and D. Wan, Eds., ed Boca Raton: CRC Press, 2007, pp. 243–274. Cited on page(s) 31, 32

[50] K. Eason, *Information technology and organizational change*. London: Taylor & Francis, 1987. Cited on page(s) 31

[51] N. Dahlback, A. Jonsson, and L. Ahrenberg, "Wizard of Oz studies: Why and how," in *IUI '93 Proceedings of the 1st international conference on Intelligent user interfaces*, New York, NY, 1993. DOI: 10.1145/169891.169968 Cited on page(s) 32

[52] A. Mihailidis, J. Boger, and A. Cavoukian, "Sensors and In-Home Collection of Health Data: A Privacy by Design Approach," Information and Privacy Commissioner Ontario & Intelligent Assistive Technology and Systems Lab, Toronto, Canada2010. Cited on page(s) 33, 35, 36

[53] J. F. Coughlin et al., "Older adult perceptions of smart home technologies: Implications for research, policy, and market innovations in healthcare," in *IEEE Proceedings of the Engineering in Medicine & Biology Confernece*, Lyon, France, 2007. DOI: 10.1109/IEMBS.2007.4352665 Cited on page(s) 33

REFERENCES 77

[54] D. Kotz, S. Avancha, and A. Baxi, "A privacy framework for mobile healt and homecare systems," in *SPIMACS'09*, Chicago, IL, 2009. DOI: 10.1145/1655084.1655086 Cited on page(s) 33

[55] J. C. Cornman, V. Freedman, and E. M. Agree, "Measurement of assistive device use: Implications for estimates of device use and disability in later life," *Gerontologist*, vol. 45, p. 347, 2005. DOI: 10.1093/geront/45.3.347 Cited on page(s) 37

[56] M. J. Scherer, T. Hart, N. Kirsch, and M. Schulthesis, "Assistive technologies for cognitive disabilities," *Critical Reviews in Physical and Rehabilitation Medicine*, vol. 17, p. 195, 2005. Cited on page(s) 37

[57] R. S. Wilson, C. F. M. de Leon, L. L. Barnes, J. A. Schneider, J. L. Bienias, D. A. Evans, and D. A. Bennett, "Participation in Cognitively Stimulating Activities and Risk of Incident Alzheimer Disease," *Journal of the American Medical Association*, vol. 287, pp. 742–748, February 2002. DOI: 10.1001/jama.287.6.742 Cited on page(s) 38

[58] A. Astell et al., "Using a touch screen computer to support relationships betweek people with dementia and caregivers," *Interacting with Computers*, vol. 22, pp. 267–275, 2010. DOI: 10.1016/j.intcom.2010.03.003 Cited on page(s) 39

[59] H. Jimison, M. Pavel, J. McKanna, and J. Pavel, "Unobtrusive monitoring of computer interactions to detect cognitive status in elders," *IEEE Trans. on Information Technology in Biomedicine*, vol. 8, pp. 248–252, 2004. DOI: 10.1109/TITB.2004.835539 Cited on page(s) 39

[60] L. C. Watson, C. L. Lewis, C. G. Moore, and D. V. Jeste, "Perceptions of depression among dementia caregivers: findings from the CATIE-AD trial," *International Journal of Geriatric Psychiatry*, vol. online, pre-print, 2010. DOI: 10.1002/gps.2539 Cited on page(s) 39

[61] R. Schulz and S. Beach, "Caregiving as a risk factor for mortality: The caregiver health effects study," *Journal of the American Medical Association*, vol. 282, pp. 2215–2219, 1999. DOI: 10.1001/jama.282.23.2215 Cited on page(s) 39

[62] J. Boger, J. Hoey, K. Fenton, T. Craig, and A. Mihailidis, "Using actors to develop technologies for older adults with dementia," *Gerontechnology*, vol. 9, pp. 450–463, 2010. DOI: 10.4017/gt.2010.09.04.001.00 Cited on page(s) 45

[63] A. J. Bharucha, V. Amand, J. Forlizzi, M. A. Dew, C. F. Reynolds, S. Stevens, and H. Wactlar, "Intelligent assistive technology applications to dementia care: Current capabilities, limitations, and future challenges," *Am J Geriatr Psychiatry*, vol. 17, pp. 88–104, 2009. DOI: 10.1097/JGP.0b013e318187dde5 Cited on page(s) 47

[64] A. M. Cook and S. M. Hussey, *Assistive Technologies: Principles and Practice*. Toronto: Mosby, 2002. Cited on page(s)

78 REFERENCES

[65] E. F. LoPresti, A. Mihailidis, and N. Kirsch, "Assistive technology for cognitive rehabilitation: State of the art," *Neuropsychological Rehabilitation,* vol. 14, pp. 5 - 39, 2004. DOI: 10.1080/09602010343000101 Cited on page(s)

[66] A. Mihailidis and G. Fernie, "Context-aware assistive devices for older adults with dementia," *Gerontechnology,* vol. 2, pp. 173 - 189, 2002. DOI: 10.4017/gt.2002.02.02.002.00 Cited on page(s) 47

[67] M. E. Pollack, "Intelligent Technology for an Aging Population: The Use of AI to Assist Elders with Cognitive Impairment," *AI Magazine,* vol. 26, pp. 9–24, Summer 2005. Cited on page(s) 48

[68] M. E. Pollack, "Autominder: A Case Study of Assistive Technology for Elders with Cognitive Impairment," *Generations: The Journal of the American Society on Aging,* vol. 30, pp. 67–69, 2006. Cited on page(s) 48, 54

[69] A. Mihailidis, J. Boger, M. Candido, and J. Hoey, "The COACH prompting system to assist older adults with dementia through handwashing: An efficacy study," *BMC Geriatrics,* vol. 8, 2008. DOI: 10.1186/1471-2318-8-28 Cited on page(s) 54

[70] J. Hoey, P. Poupart, A. von Bertoldi, T. Craig, C. Boutilier, and A. Mihailidis, "Automated Handwashing Assistance for Persons with Dementia Using video and a Partially Observable Markov Decision Process," *In Press, Computer Vision and Image Understanding, available from* http://www.computing.dundee.ac.uk/staff/jessehoey/research/coach/, 2010. DOI: 10.1016/j.cviu.2009.06.008 Cited on page(s) 54

[71] A. Mihailidis, J. Boger, M. Candido, and J. Hoey, "The COACH prompting system to assist older adults with dementia through handwashing: An efficacy study. ," *BMC Geriatrics,* vol. 8, 2008. DOI: 10.1186/1471-2318-8-28 Cited on page(s) 55

[72] J. Bauchet, S. Giroux, H. Pigot, D. Lussier-Desrochers, and Y. Lachapelle, "Pervasive assistance in smart homes for people with intellectual disabilities: A case study on meal preparation." *International Journal of Assistive Robotics and Mechatronics (IJARM),* vol. 9, pp. 42–54, 2008. Cited on page(s) 57

[73] M. Najjar, F. Courtemanche, H. Hamam, A. Dion, and J. Bauchet, "Intelligent recognition of activity of daily living for assisting memory and/or cognitively impaired elders in smart homes," *International Journal of Ambient Computing and Intelligence (IJACI),* vol. 1, pp. 46–62, 2009. DOI: 10.4018/jaci.2009062204 Cited on page(s) 57

[74] H. Kautz, L. Arnstein, G. Borriello, O. Etzioni, and a. D. Fox, "An Overview of the Assisted Cognition Project," presented at the Proc. AAAI-2002 Workshop on Automation as Caregiver: The Role of Intelligent Technology in Elder Care, 2002. Cited on page(s) 58

REFERENCES 79

[75] D. Patterson, O. Etzioni, and H. Kautz, "The Activity Compass," presented at the First International Workshop on Ubiquitous Computing for Cognitive Aids, 2002. Cited on page(s) 58

[76] L. Liao, D. Fox, and H. Kautz, "Learning and Inferring Transportation Routines," presented at the Proc Nineteenth National Conference on Artificial Intelligence (AAAI '04), San Jose, CA, 2004. DOI: 10.1016/j.artint.2007.01.006 Cited on page(s) 59

[77] R. Levinson, "A General Programming Language for Unified Planning and Control," *Artificial Intelligence: Special Issue on Planning and Scheduling*, vol. 76, July 1995. DOI: 10.1016/0004-3702(94)00075-C Cited on page(s) 59, 61

[78] J. Modayil, R. Levinson, C. Harman, D. Halper, and H. Kautz, "Integrating Sensing and Cueing for More Effective Activity Reminders," presented at the Proc. AAAI Fall 2008 Symposium on AI in Eldercare: New Solutions to Old Problems, Washington, DC, 2008. Cited on page(s) 59

[79] M. Philipose, K. P. Fishkin, D. J. Patterson, D. Fox, H. Kautz, and D. Hahnel, "Inferring activities from interactions with objects," *Pervasive Computing*, vol. 10–17, October-December 2004. DOI: 10.1109/MPRV.2004.7 Cited on page(s) 61, 62

[80] J. Lester, T. Choudhury, N. Kern, G. Borriello, and B. Hannaford, "A hybrid discriminative/generative approach for modeling human activities," presented at the Proc. IJCAI, Edinburgh, Scotland, 2005. Cited on page(s) 62

[81] W. Pentney, M. Philipose, J. A. Bilmes, and H. A. Kautz, "Learning Large Scale Common Sense Models of Everyday Life," presented at the Proceedings of AAAI, 2007. Cited on page(s) 62

[82] J. Wu, A. Osuntogun, T. Choudhury, M. Philipose, and J. M. Rehg, "A Scalable Approach to Activity Recognition Based on Object Use," presented at the Proc. of International Conference on Computer Vision (ICCV), Rio de Janeiro, Brazil, 2007. DOI: 10.1109/ICCV.2007.4408865 Cited on page(s) 62

[83] J. Hoey, B. Richards, S. Blunsden, J. Burns, T. Bartindale, D. Jackson, P. Olivier, J. N. Boger, and A. Mihailidis, "ePAD: Engaging Platform for Art Development," presented at the Working notes of the IJCAI 2009, Workshop on Intelligent Systems for Assisted Cognition, Pasadena, CA, 2009. Cited on page(s) 62, 63

[84] M. Belshaw, B. Taati, and A. Mihailidis, "Intelligent vision-based fall detection system," in *RESA-ICTA*, Toronto, Canada, 2011. Cited on page(s) 65

[85] B. Taati, J. Snoek, and A. Mihailidis, "Towards aging-in-place: Automatic assessment of product usability for older adults with dementia," in *IEEE Conference on Healthcare Informatics, Imaging, and Systems Biology*, San Jose, CA, 2011. Cited on page(s) 66

80 REFERENCES

[86] P. Lam, D. Hebert, J. Boger, H. Lacheray, D. Gardner, J. Apkarian, and A. Mihailidis, "A haptic-robotic platform for upper-limb reaching stroke therapy: Preliminary design and evaluation results," *Journal of Neuroengineering and Rehabilitation*, vol. 5, 2008. DOI: 10.1186/1743-0003-5-15 Cited on page(s) 66

[87] P. Kan, C. Boutilier, D. Hebert, J. Boger, and A. Mihailidis, "The preliminary development of a POMDP controller for upper-limb stroke rehabilitation," in *The 2nd International Conference of Technology and Aging*, Toronto, Canada, 2007. Cited on page(s) 66

[88] P. Kan, J. Hoey, and A. Mihailidis, "Stroke Rehabilitation using Haptics and a POMDP controller," presented at the (To Appear): AAAI Fall Symposium on Caring Machines: AI in Eldercare, available from http://www.computing.dundee.ac.uk/staff/jessehoey/blearn/, 2008. Cited on page(s) 66

[89] E. Lu, R. Wang, D. Hebert, J. Boger, M. Galea, and A. Mihailidis, "The development of an upper limb stroke rehabilitation robot: Identification of clinical practices and design requirements through a survey of therapists," *Disability and Rehabilitation: Assistive Technology*, 2010, in-press. DOI: 10.3109/17483107.2010.544370 Cited on page(s) 68

[90] R. Goetschalckx, P. Poupart, and J. Hoey, "Continuous correlated beta processes," in *International Joint Conference on Artificial Intelligence*, Barcelona, Spain, 2011. Cited on page(s) 68

[91] R. Huq, R. Wang, E. Lu, H. Lecheray, and A. Mihailidis, "Development of a fuzzy logic based intelligent system for autonomous guidance of post-stroke rehabilitation exercise," *IEEE Trans. on Mechatronics*, in-review. Cited on page(s) 68

[92] A. Mihailidis, P. Elinas, J. Boger, and J. Hoey, "An Intelligent Powered Wheelchair to Enable Mobility of Cognitively Impaired Older Adults: an Anticollision System," *IEEE Transactions on Neural Systems and Rehabilitation Engineering*, vol. 15, pp. 136–143, 2007. DOI: 10.1109/TNSRE.2007.891385 Cited on page(s) 71

[93] P. Viswanathan, J. Boger, J. Hoey, P. Elinas, J. Little, A. Mackworth, and A. Mihailidis, "An intelligent powered wheelchair to enable mobility in older adults with cognitively impairments," in *Robotics for Society, Cognitive Science Conference*, Vancouver, BC, 2007. Cited on page(s) 71

Authors' Biographies

ALEX MIHAILIDIS

Dr. Mihailidis is the Barbara G. Stymiest Research Chair in Rehabilitation Technology at the University of Toronto and Toronto Rehab Institute. He is an Associate Professor in the Department of Occupational Science and Occupational Therapy (U of T) and in the Institute of Biomaterials and Biomedical Engineering (U of T), with a cross appointment in the Department of Computer Science (U of T). He has been conducting research in the field of pervasive computing and intelligent systems in health for the past 13 years, having published over 100 journal papers, conference papers, and abstracts in this field. He has specifically focused on the development of intelligent home systems for elder care and wellness, technology for children with autism, and adaptive tools for nurses and clinical applications. Dr. Mihailidis is also very active in the rehabilitation engineering profession, currently as the President-Elect for RESNA (Rehabilitation Engineering and Assistive Technology Society of North America).

JENNIFER BOGER

Jennifer has been an active member in the field of computerised assistive technology for enhancing safety and independence for older adults and people with disabilities for more than eight years. Apart from advancing the technological capabilities of computer-bases assistive technologies, Jennifer's interests include the application of user-centred design to the assistive technology development process, the advancement of zero-effort technologies, and actively perusing collaboration between the diverse spectrum of stakeholders involved in the field of assistive technologies.

JESSE HOEY

Dr. Jesse Hoey is an assistant professor in the David R. Cheriton School of Computer Science at the University of Waterloo. He is also an adjunct scientist at the Toronto Rehabilitation Institute in Toronto, Canada, and an Honorary Research Fellow at the University of Dundee, Scotland. His research focuses on planning and acting in large-scale, real-world uncertain domains. He has published over 30 peer reviewed scientific papers in highly visible journals and conferences. He won the Microsoft/AAAI Distinguished Contribution Award at the 2009 IJCAI Workshop on Intelligent Systems for Assisted Cognition, for his paper on technology to facilitate creative expression in persons with dementia. He won the Best Paper award at the International Conference on Vision Systems (ICVS) in 2007 for his paper describing an assistive system for persons with dementia during hand washing. Dr. Hoey is program chair of the 2011 British Machine Vision Conference (BMVC).

TIZNEEM JIANCARO

Tizneem is a doctoral student at the University of Toronto, affiliated with the Dept. of Rehabilitation Science and the Institute of Biomaterials and Biomedical Engineering. Her background combines studies in engineering and cognitive science with work exploring the integration of human factors within design. Currently, she is interested in connections between healthcare, technology, and complex systems, and she is working on a best practices design guide to support development of technologies for Alzheimer's care.